SIMPLE
BREAD MACHINE
COOKBOOK FOR BEGINNERS

Freshly Baked Perfection

and 70 Bread Machine Recipes

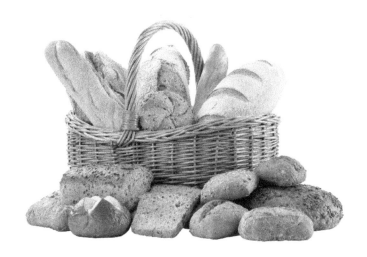

Alessia Sofia Ferrari

Simple Bread Machine Cookbook for Beginners

@2023 Alessia Sofia Ferrari

Table of Contents

BREAD MACHINE COOKBOOK

Freshly Baked Perfection

40 Irresistible Recipes for Your Bread Machine

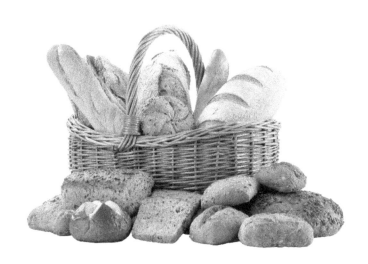

Alessia Sofia Ferrari

Bread Machine Cookbook

@2023 Alessia Sofia Ferrari

INTRODUCTION

There's something magical about the aroma of freshly baked bread wafting through the air, captivating our senses and evoking warm memories of home. In this cookbook, "Freshly Baked Perfection: 45 Irresistible Recipes for Your Bread Machine," we invite you to embark on a delightful journey into the world of bread machines, where baking delicious homemade bread becomes an effortless and rewarding experience.

The Bread Machine Revolution

Gone are the days of laborious kneading, waiting for the dough to rise, and the uncertainty of achieving that perfect loaf. The bread machine has revolutionized the art of baking, bringing the joys of homemade bread to kitchens worldwide. These compact wonders take the guesswork out of bread making, automating the entire process from mixing to baking, while leaving you with the freedom to focus on the finer things in life.

Why Choose a Bread Machine?

The answer is simple – convenience and consistency. With a bread machine by your side, you can effortlessly create a variety of breads to suit any occasion, whether it's a hearty breakfast, a wholesome family meal, or a delightful afternoon snack. From classic white loaves to specialty artisanal creations, the possibilities are endless.

The Joy of Baking at Your Fingertips

No more rushing to the bakery or settling for store-bought loaves with unknown ingredients. With "Freshly Baked Perfection," you hold the power to craft delectable, freshly baked bread whenever your heart desires. These recipes have been thoughtfully curated to cater to diverse tastes, ensuring there's something for everyone.

Our Promise to You

In this cookbook, we aim to demystify the art of bread making and instill confidence in bakers of all skill levels. Whether you're a seasoned pro or a complete novice, our step-by-step instructions will guide you through the process, ensuring consistently exceptional results every time.

Embrace the Joy of Homemade Bread

The act of baking bread carries a sense of nostalgia and tradition. It connects us to our roots and allows us to express love and care for those we share it with. So, embark on this culinary adventure with "Freshly Baked Perfection," and let the heartwarming scent of freshly baked bread fill your kitchen with love, comfort, and joy.

Get ready to experience the satisfaction of creating your very own bread masterpieces, tailored to your preferences and dietary needs. Your bread machine is a gateway to a world of flavors, textures, and creativity that will delight your taste buds and those of your loved ones. So, let's preheat those ovens, gather our ingredients, and dive into the joyous world of bread machine baking. It's time to unlock the full potential of your bread machine and create "Freshly Baked Perfection." Happy baking!

Benefits of using a bread machine for baking

Using a bread machine for baking offers numerous benefits that make it an essential kitchen appliance for bread enthusiasts. Here are some of the key advantages:

1. Time-Saving Convenience: One of the most significant benefits of a bread machine is the time it saves. Traditional bread-making involves multiple steps, including kneading, rising, and baking, which can be time-consuming. With a bread machine, you simply add the ingredients, select the appropriate settings, and let the machine do the work. This frees up your time for other activities while still allowing you to enjoy freshly baked bread.

2. Foolproof Baking: Bread machines are designed to take the guesswork out of bread-making. They have precise settings for kneading, rising, and baking, ensuring consistent and reliable results every time. Even if you're a novice baker, you can achieve professional-quality bread with minimal effort.

3. Customizable Recipes: Bread machines provide the flexibility to customize recipes according to your preferences. Whether you want to adjust the sweetness, add various grains and

seeds, or make gluten-free alternatives, the machine allows you to experiment and create personalized bread variations.

4. Freshness and Flavor: There's nothing quite like the taste and aroma of freshly baked bread. With a bread machine, you can wake up to the delightful scent of warm bread or come home to a house filled with the comforting fragrance of a just-baked loaf. Enjoying bread at its peak freshness enhances its flavor and texture, making it a delight for your taste buds.

5. Healthier Ingredients: When baking bread at home, you have complete control over the ingredients. You can choose high-quality, organic, and locally sourced ingredients, eliminating the need for artificial additives or preservatives commonly found in store-bought bread. This allows you to create healthier and more wholesome bread options for you and your family.

6. Cost-Effective: Making bread at home with a bread machine can be cost-effective in the long run. The initial investment in the machine pays off as you save money on store-bought bread, especially if you consume bread regularly.

7. Versatility: Bread machines are not limited to basic bread recipes. Many models offer additional settings for making dough for pizza, pasta, cinnamon rolls, and more. This versatility expands your baking options and encourages culinary experimentation.

8. Reduced Energy Consumption: Bread machines are designed to be energy-efficient, using considerably less energy compared to traditional ovens. This can be an eco-friendly choice for those conscious of their environmental impact.

9. Ideal for Beginners and Busy Individuals: For those new to bread-making or individuals with busy schedules, a bread machine is a game-changer. It eliminates the need for hands-on kneading and monitoring, making it a stress-free and accessible way to bake homemade bread.

In conclusion, investing in a bread machine not only simplifies the bread-making process but also empowers you to explore your creativity in the kitchen. With its time-saving convenience, consistent results, and the joy of freshly baked bread, a bread machine is a valuable addition to any home baker's arsenal.

General tips for successful bread machine baking

To ensure successful bread machine baking and achieve delicious, perfectly baked loaves, here are some general tips to keep in mind:

1. Measure Ingredients Accurately: Precise measurements are crucial for successful bread machine baking. Use measuring cups and spoons specifically designed for dry and liquid ingredients. Be mindful of using the right flour type (all-purpose, bread flour, whole wheat, etc.) as specified in the recipe.

2. Follow the Recipe: While bread machines simplify the process, it's essential to follow the recipe instructions carefully. Each bread machine model may have specific requirements for ingredient order and settings.

3. Use Fresh Ingredients: For the best results, use fresh and high-quality ingredients. Check the expiration date of yeast, baking powder, and other leavening agents, as expired ingredients can affect the bread's rise and flavor.

4. Adjust Liquid and Flour Ratios: Depending on factors like humidity and altitude, you may need to adjust the amount of liquid or flour in the recipe. The dough should form a smooth ball without being too sticky or dry.

5. Avoid Overmixing: Overmixing the dough can lead to tough bread. Let the bread machine handle the mixing and kneading process. Avoid opening the lid during these phases to ensure the best texture.

6. Add Mix-ins at the Right Time: If your recipe includes mix-ins like nuts, seeds, dried fruits, or chocolate chips, add them

at the appropriate time during the baking cycle. Many bread machines have an alert for adding mix-ins.

7. Check Dough Consistency: During the kneading phase, peek inside the bread machine to ensure the dough isn't too dry or too wet. Adjust with additional liquid or flour if needed to achieve the ideal consistency.

8. Grease the Bread Pan: To prevent sticking, lightly grease the bread pan before adding the ingredients. This will also make it easier to remove the finished loaf.

9. Be Mindful of Yeast Placement: When using delayed start settings, ensure the yeast does not come into contact with the liquid prematurely. Place the yeast on top of the flour to keep it dry until the machine starts.

10. Use Room Temperature Ingredients: Bring eggs, milk, and other refrigerated ingredients to room temperature before adding them to the bread machine. This helps with proper yeast activation and even baking.

11. Select the Right Settings: Choose the appropriate setting for the type of bread you're making. Most bread machines have settings for basic white bread, whole wheat, sweet bread, and more.

12. Remove the Bread Promptly: Once the bread is done baking, promptly remove it from the machine to prevent it from becoming soggy due to the residual heat.

13. Let It Cool: Allow the bread to cool on a wire rack for at least 20-30 minutes before slicing. Cutting the bread too soon can result in a gummy texture.

With these tips, you'll be well on your way to mastering the art of bread machine baking and enjoying a delightful array of freshly baked bread right from the comfort of your home.

Overview of essential ingredients and equipment

To achieve successful bread machine baking and create delicious loaves, you'll need essential ingredients and equipment. Here's an overview of what you'll require:

Essential Ingredients:

- Flour: The foundation of any bread recipe. Common options include all-purpose flour, bread flour (higher protein content for better structure), whole wheat flour (for nuttier flavor and added nutrition), and specialty flours like rye or spelt.

- Yeast: Responsible for fermentation and leavening the dough. Active dry yeast or instant yeast are commonly used in bread machine recipes. Make sure it's fresh and within its expiration date for optimal results.
- Liquid: Usually water, milk, or a combination of both. It activates the yeast and helps bind the ingredients. Depending on the recipe, other liquids like fruit juice, buttermilk, or yogurt may be used.
- Sweetener: Adds flavor and helps with browning. Common sweeteners include sugar, honey, maple syrup, or molasses. Some recipes might use alternative sweeteners like agave nectar or stevia.
- Fat: Contributes to the bread's tenderness and flavor. Common fats include butter, vegetable oil, olive oil, or coconut oil.
- Salt: Enhances the bread's flavor and controls yeast activity. It's an essential ingredient for proper bread development.
- Extras: Depending on the recipe, you might add ingredients like eggs, herbs, spices, nuts, seeds, dried fruits, or chocolate chips to create specialty bread varieties.

Equipment:

- Bread Machine: The star of the show! Choose a reliable bread machine with settings that suit your baking needs. Some machines have more advanced features like gluten-free settings, crust color options, and delay start timers.

- Measuring Cups and Spoons: Accurate measurements are crucial for successful baking. Invest in a set of dry and liquid measuring cups and spoons.
- Mixing Bowl: While the bread machine handles the mixing and kneading, you might need a mixing bowl for some recipes that require additional hand mixing.
- Bread Pans: Most bread machines come with a removable bread pan. Ensure it's clean and properly greased before adding the ingredients.
- Cooling Rack: After baking, allow the bread to cool on a wire cooling rack to avoid condensation and maintain the crust's texture.

- Oven Mitts or Kitchen Towels: Bread machine pans and freshly baked bread can be hot. Protect your hands with oven mitts or kitchen towels when handling them.
- Bread Knife or Slicer: For perfectly even slices, use a bread knife or slicer when the loaf has cooled.

With these essential ingredients and equipment, you're ready to dive into the world of bread machine baking and create a variety of delightful breads to satisfy your cravings and impress your loved ones.

Happy baking!

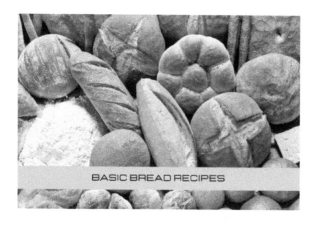

BASIC BREAD RECIPES

Classic White Bread

Ingredients:

- 1 cup warm water (about 110°F/43°C)
- 2 tablespoons granulated sugar
- 1 1/2 teaspoons active dry yeast
- 3 cups all-purpose flour
- 2 tablespoons unsalted butter, softened
- 1 1/2 teaspoons salt

Instructions:

1. In a small bowl, combine warm water and sugar. Stir until the sugar is dissolved. Sprinkle the active dry yeast over the water and let it sit for about 5 minutes or until it becomes frothy.
2. In the bread machine pan, add the flour, softened butter, and salt. Pour the yeast mixture over the flour.

3. Place the bread machine pan into the bread machine and set it to the "Basic" or "White Bread" cycle. Select the desired loaf size (usually 1 or 1.5 pounds) and crust color (light, medium, or dark) according to your preference.
4. Close the lid and start the bread machine. The machine will begin mixing, kneading, and rising the dough.
5. Once the bread machine completes the cycle and the bread is baked, carefully remove the bread pan from the machine using oven mitts or kitchen towels.
6. Allow the bread to cool in the pan for a few minutes before transferring it to a wire rack to cool completely.
7. Once cooled, slice the bread and enjoy!

Note:

For a softer crust, brush the top of the bread with melted butter immediately after baking. You can add variations to this classic white bread recipe by incorporating ingredients like milk powder, a touch of honey, or even dried herbs to customize the flavor to your liking.

This classic white bread is perfect for sandwiches, toasts, or simply enjoyed with a spread of butter. With your bread machine doing the hard work, you can relish the comforting taste of homemade bread without the fuss.

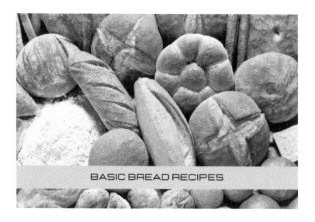

Whole Wheat Bread

Ingredients:

- 1 1/4 cups warm water (about 110°F/43°C)
- 2 tablespoons honey or molasses (for sweetness)
- 2 tablespoons vegetable oil or melted butter
- 1 1/2 teaspoons active dry yeast
- 3 cups whole wheat flour
- 1 teaspoon salt

Optional Add-ins:

- 1/4 cup rolled oats or wheat bran for added texture
- 2 tablespoons ground flaxseed for extra nutrition
- 1/4 cup nuts or seeds for a nutty crunch (e.g., sunflower seeds or chopped walnuts

Instructions:

1. In a small bowl, combine warm water and honey or molasses. Stir until the sweetener is dissolved. Sprinkle the active dry yeast over the water and let it sit for about 5 minutes or until it becomes frothy.
2. In the bread machine pan, add the whole wheat flour and salt. If using, add the optional rolled oats or wheat bran and ground flaxseed.
3. Pour the yeast mixture and vegetable oil or melted butter over the flour. If adding nuts or seeds, sprinkle them on top.
4. Place the bread machine pan into the bread machine and set it to the "Whole Wheat" or "Whole Grain" cycle. Select the desired loaf size (usually 1 or 1.5 pounds) and crust color (light, medium, or dark) according to your preference.
5. Close the lid and start the bread machine. The machine will begin mixing, kneading, and rising the dough.
6. Once the bread machine completes the cycle and the bread is baked, carefully remove the bread pan from the machine using oven mitts or kitchen towels.
7. Allow the bread to cool in the pan for a few minutes before transferring it to a wire rack to cool completely.
8. Once cooled, slice the whole wheat bread and enjoy!

Note:

This whole wheat bread is naturally dense and hearty. For a softer texture, you can add a small amount of all-purpose flour to the whole wheat flour (about 1/2 cup) to lighten the loaf. Feel free to customize the recipe with different seeds, nuts, or dried fruits to add variety and personal touches to your whole wheat bread.

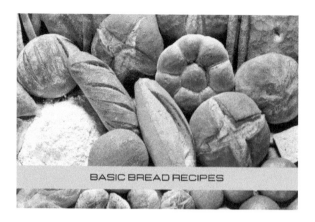

Multigrain Bread

Ingredients:

- 1 1/4 cups warm water (about 110°F/43°C)
- 2 tablespoons honey or maple syrup (for sweetness)
- 2 tablespoons vegetable oil or melted butter
- 1 1/2 teaspoons active dry yeast
- 1 cup whole wheat flour
- 1/2 cup bread flour
- 1/2 cup rye flour
- 1/2 cup rolled oats
- 1/4 cup cornmeal
- 1/4 cup flaxseeds or sesame seeds
- 1 teaspoon salt

Optional Add-ins:

- 1/4 cup sunflower seeds or pumpkin seeds for extra crunch
- 1/4 cup dried fruits (e.g., cranberries or raisins) for a touch of sweetness
- 1/4 teaspoon ground cinnamon for warm, aromatic flavor

Instructions:

1. In a small bowl, combine warm water and honey or maple syrup. Stir until the sweetener is dissolved. Sprinkle the active dry yeast over the water and let it sit for about 5 minutes or until it becomes frothy.
2. In the bread machine pan, add the whole wheat flour, bread flour, rye flour, rolled oats, cornmeal, flaxseeds or sesame seeds, and salt.
3. If using any optional add-ins, add them to the dry ingredients.
4. Pour the yeast mixture and vegetable oil or melted butter over the dry ingredients.
5. Place the bread machine pan into the bread machine and set it to the "Multigrain" or "Whole Grain" cycle. Select the desired loaf size (usually 1 or 1.5 pounds) and crust color (light, medium, or dark) according to your preference.
6. Close the lid and start the bread machine. The machine will begin mixing, kneading, and rising the multigrain dough.
7. Once the bread machine completes the cycle and the bread is baked, carefully remove the bread pan from the machine using oven mitts or kitchen towels.
8. Allow the multigrain bread to cool in the pan for a few minutes before transferring it to a wire rack to cool completely.
9. Once cooled, slice the multigrain bread and relish the wholesome goodness!

Note:

This multigrain bread is packed with nutritious seeds, grains, and fibers. You can tailor it to your taste by adding or omitting ingredients based on your preferences. For a touch of sweetness and flavor, consider using the optional dried fruits and ground cinnamon.

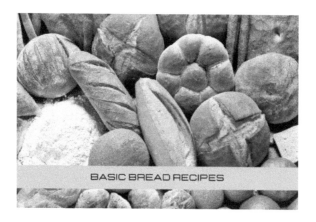

BASIC BREAD RECIPES

Honey Oat Bread

Ingredients:

- 1 1/4 cups warm water (about 110°F/43°C)
- 2 tablespoons honey
- 2 tablespoons vegetable oil or melted butter
- 1 1/2 teaspoons active dry yeast
- 1 cup bread flour
- 1 cup whole wheat flour
- 1/2 cup rolled oats
- 1 1/2 teaspoons salt

Optional Add-ins:

- 2 tablespoons sunflower seeds or chopped nuts for extra crunch and flavor
- 1/4 cup raisins or dried cranberries for a hint of sweetness
- 1/2 teaspoon ground cinnamon for warm, aromatic notes

Instructions:

1. In a small bowl, combine warm water and honey. Stir until the honey is dissolved. Sprinkle the active dry yeast over the water and let it sit for about 5 minutes or until it becomes frothy.
2. In the bread machine pan, add the bread flour, whole wheat flour, rolled oats, and salt.
3. If using any optional add-ins, such as sunflower seeds, nuts, raisins, or ground cinnamon, add them to the dry ingredients.
4. Pour the yeast mixture and vegetable oil or melted butter over the dry ingredients.
5. Place the bread machine pan into the bread machine and set it to the "Basic" or "Whole Wheat" cycle. Select the desired loaf size (usually 1 or 1.5 pounds) and crust color (light, medium, or dark) according to your preference.
6. Close the lid and start the bread machine. The machine will begin mixing, kneading, and rising the honey oat dough.
7. Once the bread machine completes the cycle and the bread is baked, carefully remove the bread pan from the machine using oven mitts or kitchen towels.
8. Allow the Honey Oat Bread to cool in the pan for a few minutes before transferring it to a wire rack to cool completely.
9. Once cooled, slice the bread and enjoy the delightful sweetness of honey and the wholesome texture of oats!

Note:

This Honey Oat Bread is a perfect balance of sweetness and heartiness. You can customize it by adding your favorite nuts, seeds, or dried fruits. The optional ground cinnamon adds a warm, comforting aroma and flavor to the bread.

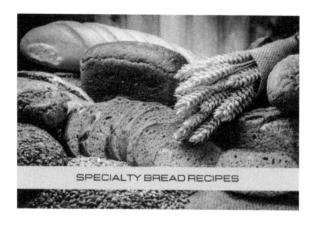

Cinnamon Swirl Bread

Ingredients for the Bread:

- 1 cup warm milk (about 110°F/43°C)
- 2 tablespoons unsalted butter, softened
- 3 cups bread flour
- 2 tablespoons granulated sugar
- 1 1/2 teaspoons active dry yeast
- 1 teaspoon salt

For the Cinnamon Swirl:

- 1/4 cup granulated sugar
- 2 teaspoons ground cinnamon

For the Glaze (Optional):

- 1/2 cup powdered sugar
- 1-2 tablespoons milk or water
- 1/2 teaspoon vanilla extract

Instructions:

1. In a small bowl, combine warm milk and softened butter. Stir until the butter is melted.

2. In the bread machine pan, add bread flour, sugar, active dry yeast, and salt.
3. Pour the milk and butter mixture over the dry ingredients in the bread machine pan.
4. Place the bread machine pan into the bread machine and set it to the "Dough" or "Basic" cycle. Start the machine to mix and knead the dough.
5. While the dough is kneading, prepare the cinnamon swirl mixture by mixing granulated sugar and ground cinnamon in a separate bowl.
6. Once the dough cycle is complete, remove the dough from the bread machine and place it on a lightly floured surface.
7. Roll out the dough into a rectangular shape using a rolling pin. Sprinkle the cinnamon swirl mixture evenly over the rolled-out dough.
8. Carefully roll up the dough from the shorter end, creating a cinnamon swirl log.
9. Place the cinnamon swirl log into a greased loaf pan. Cover the pan with a clean kitchen towel and let the dough rise for about 30-45 minutes or until it doubles in size.
10. Preheat your oven to 350°F (175°C) while the dough is rising.
11. Once the dough has risen, bake the Cinnamon Swirl Bread in the preheated oven for approximately 30-35 minutes or until it turns golden brown.
12. If desired, prepare the glaze by mixing powdered sugar, milk or water, and vanilla extract. Drizzle the glaze over the cooled bread.
13. Allow the bread to cool in the pan for a few minutes before transferring it to a wire rack to cool completely.
14. Slice the Cinnamon Swirl Bread and enjoy the delightful flavors and swirls of cinnamon goodness!

Note: You can add chopped nuts or raisins to the cinnamon swirl mixture for extra texture and flavor. For a more pronounced cinnamon flavor, you can increase the amount of ground cinnamon in the swirl mixture.

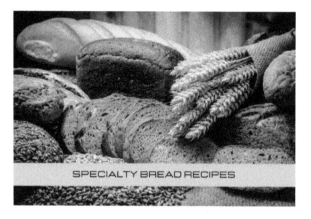

SPECIALTY BREAD RECIPES

Sunflower Seed Bread

Ingredients:

- 1 cup warm water (about 110°F/43°C)
- 2 tablespoons honey or maple syrup (for sweetness)
- 2 tablespoons vegetable oil or melted butter
- 1 1/2 teaspoons active dry yeast
- 2 1/2 cups bread flour
- 1/2 cup whole wheat flour
- 1/2 cup rolled oats
- 1/4 cup sunflower seeds (plus extra for topping)
- 1 1/2 teaspoons salt

Instructions:

1. In a small bowl, combine warm water and honey or maple syrup. Stir until the sweetener is dissolved. Sprinkle the active dry yeast over the water and let it sit for about 5 minutes or until it becomes frothy.

2. In the bread machine pan, add the bread flour, whole wheat flour, rolled oats, sunflower seeds, and salt.
3. Pour the yeast mixture and vegetable oil or melted butter over the dry ingredients.
4. Place the bread machine pan into the bread machine and set it to the "Basic" or "Whole Wheat" cycle. Select the desired loaf size (usually 1 or 1.5 pounds) and crust color (light, medium, or dark) according to your preference.
5. Close the lid and start the bread machine. The machine will begin mixing, kneading, and rising the sunflower seed bread dough.
6. Once the bread machine completes the cycle and the bread is baked, carefully remove the bread pan from the machine using oven mitts or kitchen towels.
7. While the bread is still warm, brush the top with water and sprinkle additional sunflower seeds for a delightful presentation.
8. Allow the Sunflower Seed Bread to cool in the pan for a few minutes before transferring it to a wire rack to cool completely.
9. Once cooled, slice the bread and savor the nutty goodness of sunflower seeds!

Note:

For an extra nutty flavor, lightly toast the sunflower seeds before adding them to the dough. Sunflower Seed Bread is perfect for toasting and can be enjoyed with various spreads or used as the base for sandwiches.

Indulge in the rich, nutty flavor and crunch of this homemade Sunflower Seed Bread, perfect for breakfast, lunch, or as a delicious snack. With the bread machine simplifying the process, you can relish the joy of freshly baked bread with wholesome sunflower seeds to delight your taste buds.

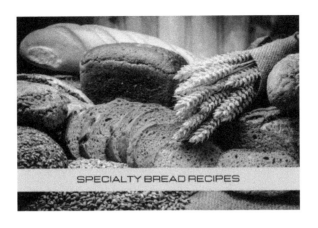

SPECIALTY BREAD RECIPES

Rosemary & Olive Oil Bread

Ingredients:

- 1 cup warm water (about 110°F/43°C)
- 2 tablespoons olive oil
- 1 1/2 teaspoons active dry yeast
- 3 cups bread flour
- 1 tablespoon granulated sugar
- 1 1/2 teaspoons dried rosemary (crushed) or 1 tablespoon fresh rosemary (finely chopped)
- 1 teaspoon salt
- 1/2 cup pitted and chopped black olives (such as Kalamata olives) or green olives (optional)

Instructions:

1. In a small bowl, combine warm water and olive oil.
2. In the bread machine pan, add bread flour, sugar, dried or fresh rosemary, and salt.
3. Pour the olive oil and water mixture over the dry ingredients.
4. Sprinkle the active dry yeast over the liquids.
5. If using olives, add the chopped olives to the bread machine pan.

6. Place the bread machine pan into the bread machine and set it to the "Dough" or "Basic" cycle. Start the machine to mix and knead the dough.
7. While the dough is kneading, check the consistency. If the dough appears too dry, add a tablespoon of water at a time until the dough forms a smooth ball. If it's too sticky, add a tablespoon of flour at a time.
8. Once the dough cycle is complete, remove the dough from the bread machine and place it on a lightly floured surface.
9. Shape the dough into a loaf or place it into a greased loaf pan for a traditional loaf shape.
10. Cover the loaf with a clean kitchen towel and let it rise for about 30-45 minutes or until it doubles in size.
11. Preheat your oven to 375°F (190°C) while the dough is rising.
12. Once the dough has risen, slash the top of the loaf with a sharp knife to create decorative cuts.
13. Bake the Rosemary & Olive Oil Bread in the preheated oven for approximately 25-30 minutes or until it turns golden brown and sounds hollow when tapped.
14. Allow the bread to cool in the pan or on a wire rack before slicing and savoring the aromatic goodness!

Note: For added flavor, you can infuse the olive oil with rosemary by heating it gently in a saucepan with fresh rosemary sprigs, then letting it cool before using it in the recipe. This Rosemary & Olive Oil Bread is perfect for serving with olive oil and balsamic vinegar for dipping.

Indulge in the savory and herb-infused delight of this homemade Rosemary & Olive Oil Bread, perfect for elevating your meals and impressing your guests. With the bread machine simplifying the process, you can enjoy the enchanting flavors and aroma of freshly baked bread in no time.

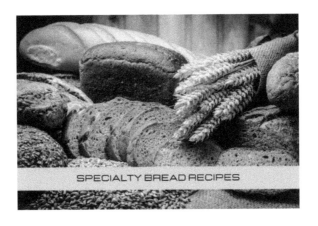

SPECIALTY BREAD RECIPES

Jalapeno Cheddar Bread

Ingredients:

- 1 cup warm water (about 110°F/43°C)
- 2 tablespoons vegetable oil or melted butter
- 1 1/2 teaspoons active dry yeast
- 3 cups bread flour
- 1 teaspoon salt
- 1 cup shredded cheddar cheese (mild or sharp, based on preference)
- 2-3 fresh jalapeno peppers, seeds removed and finely chopped (adjust to your desired level of spiciness)

Instructions:

1. In a small bowl, combine warm water and vegetable oil or melted butter.
2. In the bread machine pan, add bread flour and salt.
3. Pour the water and oil mixture over the dry ingredients.
4. Sprinkle the active dry yeast over the liquids.
5. Add the shredded cheddar cheese and chopped jalapeno peppers to the bread machine pan.

6. Place the bread machine pan into the bread machine and set it to the "Dough" or "Basic" cycle. Start the machine to mix and knead the dough.
7. While the dough is kneading, check the consistency. If the dough appears too dry, add a tablespoon of water at a time until the dough forms a smooth ball. If it's too sticky, add a tablespoon of flour at a time.
8. Once the dough cycle is complete, remove the dough from the bread machine and place it on a lightly floured surface.
9. Shape the dough into a loaf or place it into a greased loaf pan for a traditional loaf shape.
10. Cover the loaf with a clean kitchen towel and let it rise for about 30-45 minutes or until it doubles in size.
11. Preheat your oven to 375°F (190°C) while the dough is rising.
12. Once the dough has risen, slash the top of the loaf with a sharp knife to create decorative cuts.
13. Bake the Jalapeno Cheddar Bread in the preheated oven for approximately 25-30 minutes or until it turns golden brown and sounds hollow when tapped.
14. Allow the bread to cool in the pan or on a wire rack before slicing and savoring the flavorful and slightly spicy goodness!

Note:

If you prefer a milder spiciness, you can remove the seeds and membranes from the jalapeno peppers before chopping them. This Jalapeno Cheddar Bread is perfect for sandwiches, grilled cheese, or enjoyed on its own.

Indulge in the bold flavors and spicy charm of this homemade Jalapeno Cheddar Bread, perfect for adding excitement to your meals and gatherings. With the bread machine streamlining the process, you can enjoy the deliciousness of freshly baked bread with a delightful kick.

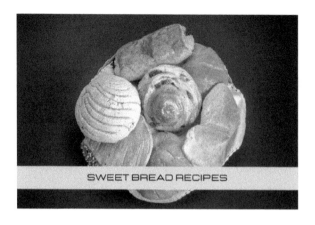

Cinnamon Raisin Bread

Ingredients:

- 1 cup warm milk (about 110°F/43°C)
- 2 tablespoons unsalted butter, softened
- 1/4 cup granulated sugar
- 1 1/2 teaspoons active dry yeast
- 3 cups bread flour
- 1 teaspoon ground cinnamon
- 1/2 teaspoon salt
- 1/2 cup raisins (dark or golden, based on preference)

For the Cinnamon Swirl:

- 2 tablespoons unsalted butter, softened
- 1/4 cup packed light brown sugar
- 1 teaspoon ground cinnamon

Optional Glaze:

- 1/2 cup powdered sugar
- 1-2 tablespoons milk or water
- 1/2 teaspoon vanilla extract

Instructions:

1. In a small bowl, combine warm milk, softened butter, and granulated sugar. Stir until the sugar is dissolved. Sprinkle the active dry yeast over the mixture and let it sit for about 5 minutes or until it becomes frothy.
2. In the bread machine pan, add bread flour, ground cinnamon, and salt.
3. Pour the milk mixture and yeast over the dry ingredients in the bread machine pan.
4. Set your bread machine to the "Dough" or "Basic" cycle. Start the machine to mix and knead the dough.
5. While the dough is kneading, prepare the cinnamon swirl mixture. In a separate bowl, mix together softened butter, brown sugar, and ground cinnamon until well combined.
6. Once the dough cycle is complete, remove the dough from the bread machine and place it on a lightly floured surface.
7. Roll out the dough into a rectangular shape using a rolling pin.
8. Spread the cinnamon swirl mixture evenly over the rolled-out dough, and then sprinkle the raisins on top.
9. Carefully roll up the dough from the shorter end, creating a cinnamon swirl log.
10. Place the cinnamon swirl log into a greased loaf pan. Cover the pan with a clean kitchen towel and let the dough rise for about 30-45 minutes or until it doubles in size.
11. Preheat your oven to 375°F (190°C) while the dough is rising.
12. Once the dough has risen, bake the Cinnamon Raisin Bread in the preheated oven for approximately 25-30 minutes or until it turns golden brown and sounds hollow when tapped.
13. If desired, prepare the glaze by mixing powdered sugar, milk or water, and vanilla extract. Drizzle the glaze over the cooled bread.

14. Allow the bread to cool in the pan for a few minutes before transferring it to a wire rack to cool completely.
15. Slice the Cinnamon Raisin Bread and enjoy!

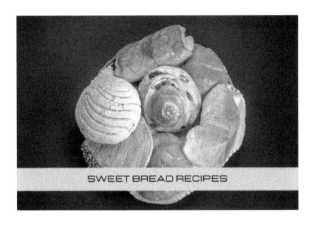

SWEET BREAD RECIPES

Lemon Poppy Seed Bread

Ingredients:

- 1 cup warm milk (about 110°F/43°C)
- 2 tablespoons unsalted butter, softened
- 1/2 cup granulated sugar
- Zest of 2 lemons
- 1 1/2 teaspoons active dry yeast
- 3 cups bread flour
- 1 tablespoon poppy seeds
- 1/2 teaspoon salt
- 2 tablespoons freshly squeezed lemon juice

Optional Glaze:

- 1/2 cup powdered sugar
- 2 tablespoons freshly squeezed lemon juice

Instructions:

1. In a small bowl, combine warm milk, softened butter, granulated sugar, and lemon zest. Stir until the sugar is

dissolved. Sprinkle the active dry yeast over the mixture and let it sit for about 5 minutes or until it becomes frothy.

2. In the bread machine pan, add bread flour, poppy seeds, and salt.
3. Pour the milk mixture and yeast over the dry ingredients in the bread machine pan.
4. Set your bread machine to the "Dough" or "Basic" cycle. Start the machine to mix and knead the dough.
5. While the dough is kneading, preheat your oven to 375°F (190°C).
6. Once the dough cycle is complete, remove the dough from the bread machine and place it on a lightly floured surface.
7. Shape the dough into a loaf or place it into a greased loaf pan for a traditional loaf shape.
8. Cover the loaf with a clean kitchen towel and let it rise for about 30-45 minutes or until it doubles in size.
9. Using a sharp knife, make a few shallow slashes on top of the risen loaf for a decorative touch.
10. Bake the Lemon Poppy Seed Bread in the preheated oven for approximately 25-30 minutes or until it turns golden brown and sounds hollow when tapped.
11. While the bread is baking, prepare the optional glaze by mixing powdered sugar and freshly squeezed lemon juice until smooth.
12. Once the bread is baked, remove it from the oven and let it cool in the pan for a few minutes before transferring it to a wire rack to cool completely.
13. Drizzle the lemon glaze over the cooled Lemon Poppy Seed Bread for extra lemony goodness.
14. Slice the bread and enjoy the delightful citrus flavors and crunch of poppy seeds!

Note:

If you prefer a less intense lemon flavor, you can reduce the amount of lemon zest and lemon juice. Lemon Poppy Seed Bread is perfect for breakfast or as a delightful afternoon snack.

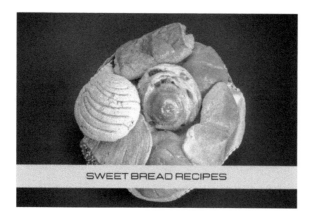

Cranberry Orange Bread

Ingredients:

- 1 cup warm milk (about 110°F/43°C)
- 2 tablespoons unsalted butter, softened
- 1/2 cup granulated sugar
- Zest of 1 orange
- 1 1/2 teaspoons active dry yeast
- 3 cups bread flour
- 1 teaspoon salt
- 1/2 cup dried cranberries
- 2 tablespoons freshly squeezed orange juice

Optional Glaze:

- 1/2 cup powdered sugar
- 2 tablespoons freshly squeezed orange juice

Instructions:

1. In a small bowl, combine warm milk, softened butter, granulated sugar, and orange zest. Stir until the sugar is dissolved. Sprinkle the active dry yeast over the mixture and let it sit for about 5 minutes or until it becomes frothy.
2. In the bread machine pan, add bread flour and salt.

3. Pour the milk mixture and yeast over the dry ingredients in the bread machine pan.
4. Set your bread machine to the "Dough" or "Basic" cycle. Start the machine to mix and knead the dough.
5. While the dough is kneading, preheat your oven to 375°F (190°C).
6. Once the dough cycle is complete, remove the dough from the bread machine and place it on a lightly floured surface.
7. Knead in the dried cranberries and freshly squeezed orange juice into the dough until evenly distributed.
8. Shape the dough into a loaf or place it into a greased loaf pan for a traditional loaf shape.
9. Cover the loaf with a clean kitchen towel and let it rise for about 30-45 minutes or until it doubles in size.
10. Using a sharp knife, make a few shallow slashes on top of the risen loaf for a decorative touch.
11. Bake the Cranberry Orange Bread in the preheated oven for approximately 25-30 minutes or until it turns golden brown and sounds hollow when tapped.
12. While the bread is baking, prepare the optional glaze by mixing powdered sugar and freshly squeezed orange juice until smooth.
13. Once the bread is baked, remove it from the oven and let it cool in the pan for a few minutes before transferring it to a wire rack to cool completely.
14. Drizzle the orange glaze over the cooled Cranberry Orange Bread for extra citrusy sweetness.
15. Slice the bread and enjoy the delightful combination of cranberries and oranges!

Note:

If you prefer a less intense orange flavor, you can reduce the amount of orange zest and orange juice. Cranberry Orange Bread is perfect for breakfast or as a lovely addition to your holiday gatherings.

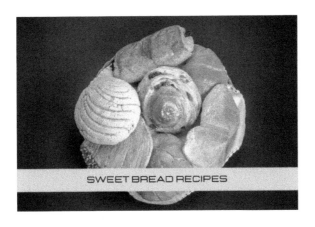

SWEET BREAD RECIPES

Apple Cinnamon Bread

Ingredients:

- 1 cup warm milk (about 110°F/43°C)
- 2 tablespoons unsalted butter, softened
- 1/2 cup granulated sugar
- 1 1/2 teaspoons active dry yeast
- 3 cups bread flour
- 1 teaspoon ground cinnamon
- 1/2 teaspoon salt
- 1 cup peeled and finely chopped apples (such as Granny Smith or Honeycrisp)
- 1/2 cup chopped walnuts or pecans (optional, for added crunch)

Instructions:

1. In a small bowl, combine warm milk, softened butter, and granulated sugar. Stir until the sugar is dissolved. Sprinkle the active dry yeast over the mixture and let it sit for about 5 minutes or until it becomes frothy.
2. In the bread machine pan, add bread flour, ground cinnamon, and salt.

45

3. Pour the milk mixture and yeast over the dry ingredients in the bread machine pan.
4. Set your bread machine to the "Dough" or "Basic" cycle. Start the machine to mix and knead the dough.
5. While the dough is kneading, preheat your oven to 375°F (190°C).
6. Once the dough cycle is complete, remove the dough from the bread machine and place it on a lightly floured surface.
7. Knead in the chopped apples and chopped walnuts or pecans (if using) into the dough until evenly distributed.
8. Shape the dough into a loaf or place it into a greased loaf pan for a traditional loaf shape.
9. Cover the loaf with a clean kitchen towel and let it rise for about 30-45 minutes or until it doubles in size.
10. Using a sharp knife, make a few shallow slashes on top of the risen loaf for a decorative touch.
11. Bake the Apple Cinnamon Bread in the preheated oven for approximately 25-30 minutes or until it turns golden brown and sounds hollow when tapped.
12. Allow the bread to cool in the pan for a few minutes before transferring it to a wire rack to cool completely.
13. Slice the bread and enjoy the delightful combination of apples and cinnamon!

Note:

If you prefer a sweeter bread, you can sprinkle a little bit of granulated sugar on top of the loaf before baking. Apple Cinnamon Bread is perfect for breakfast or as a tasty afternoon snack.

Indulge in the comforting and aromatic goodness of this homemade Apple Cinnamon Bread, perfect for bringing the flavors of fall to your table. With the bread machine taking care of the kneading and rising, you can savor the joy of freshly baked bread with the delightful combination of apples and cinnamon.

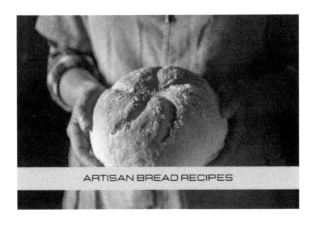

ARTISAN BREAD RECIPES

Sourdough Bread

Ingredients For the Starter (Leaven):

- 50g active sourdough starter (100% hydration)
- 100g bread flour
- 100g water (room temperature)

For the Dough:

- 400g bread flour
- 240g water (room temperature)
- 9g salt

Instructions:

1. Preparing the Starter (Leaven):
2. In a medium-sized bowl, mix the sourdough starter, bread flour, and water until well combined.
3. Cover the bowl with a clean kitchen towel or plastic wrap and let it sit at room temperature for about 4-6 hours or until the leaven is bubbly and has doubled in size.

Making the Dough:

1. In a large mixing bowl, combine 400g of bread flour and 240g of water. Mix until all the flour is hydrated, cover,

and let it rest for 30 minutes. This step is called the autolyse and helps improve the dough's extensibility.

2. After the autolyse, add the leaven to the dough and mix it in, incorporating it thoroughly.

3. Add the salt to the dough and mix until well combined. You can use your hands or a dough scraper.

4. Perform a series of stretch and folds to strengthen the dough. Do this by grabbing one edge of the dough, stretching it upward, and then folding it back onto the dough. Rotate the bowl and repeat this process three or four times.

5. Cover the bowl with a kitchen towel or plastic wrap and let the dough rest for about 30 minutes.

6. Perform another set of stretch and folds, cover the bowl, and let it rest for 30 minutes.

7. Repeat the stretch and folds two more times, letting the dough rest for 30 minutes between each set.

8. After the final set of stretch and folds, cover the bowl and let the dough bulk ferment at room temperature for about 4-6 hours. During this time, the dough should rise and develop air pockets.

9. After bulk fermentation, shape the dough into a boule (round loaf) or batard (oval loaf). You can use a bench scraper to help shape the dough.

10. Place the shaped dough into a floured banneton or a bowl lined with a floured kitchen towel, seam-side up.

11. Cover the dough with a kitchen towel or a plastic bag and let it undergo the final proofing in the refrigerator for 8-12 hours or overnight.

Baking the Sourdough Bread:

1. Preheat your oven to 450°F (230°C) with a Dutch oven or a baking stone placed inside. If using a Dutch oven, preheat it along with the oven.

2. Carefully remove the dough from the refrigerator and score the top with a sharp knife or a bread lame.

3. If using a Dutch oven, carefully place the dough into the preheated Dutch oven, cover it with the lid, and bake for 20 minutes. Then, remove the lid and continue baking for another 20-25 minutes or until the bread is golden brown.
4. If using a baking stone, gently slide the dough onto the hot baking stone and bake for 30-35 minutes or until the bread is golden brown.
5. Once the bread is baked, remove it from the oven and let it cool on a wire rack for at least an hour before slicing.

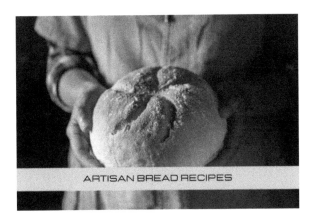

ARTISAN BREAD RECIPES

Ciabatta Bread

Ingredients:

- 500g bread flour
- 400g water (room temperature)
- 10g salt
- 5g active dry yeast
- 2 tablespoons olive oil (plus extra for greasing)

Instructions:

1. In a large mixing bowl, combine bread flour and water. Stir until all the flour is hydrated, cover the bowl, and let it rest for about 30 minutes. This step is called the autolyse and helps improve the dough's extensibility.

49

2. After the autolyse, add the salt and active dry yeast to the dough. Mix until everything is well combined.
3. Add the olive oil to the dough and knead it until the oil is fully incorporated. The dough will be sticky and wet.
4. Perform a series of stretch and folds to develop the gluten in the dough. Do this by grabbing one edge of the dough, stretching it upward, and then folding it back onto the dough. Rotate the bowl and repeat this process several times.
5. Cover the bowl with a kitchen towel or plastic wrap and let the dough bulk ferment at room temperature for about 1.5 to 2 hours. During this time, perform a set of stretch and folds every 30 minutes for the first 1.5 hours.
6. After bulk fermentation, lightly flour your work surface and gently turn out the dough. Be careful not to deflate the dough too much.
7. Divide the dough into two or three equal portions, depending on the size of ciabatta loaves you desire.
8. Shape each portion into an elongated, oval loaf, being gentle to preserve the air bubbles within the dough.
9. Transfer the shaped loaves to a well-floured surface or a floured couche (a fabric used for proofing dough).
10. Cover the loaves with a kitchen towel and let them undergo the final proofing for about 1 to 1.5 hours, or until they have visibly expanded and feel airy to the touch.
11. While the loaves are proofing, preheat your oven to 450°F (230°C) and place a baking stone or an inverted baking sheet on the middle rack.
12. Carefully transfer the proofed loaves onto a parchment-lined peel or an inverted baking sheet for easy transfer to the oven.
13. Slide the loaves onto the preheated baking stone or baking sheet and bake for about 20-25 minutes, or until the ciabatta loaves are golden brown and have a crisp crust.

14. Remove the ciabatta loaves from the oven and let them cool on a wire rack.

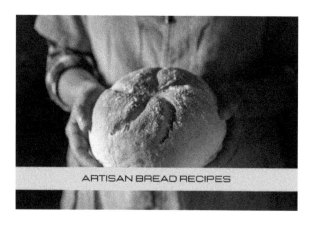

ARTISAN BREAD RECIPES

Focaccia Bread

Ingredients:

- 500g bread flour
- 400ml lukewarm water
- 10g salt
- 7g active dry yeast
- 60ml extra-virgin olive oil (plus extra for drizzling)
- 1-2 tablespoons dried Italian herbs (such as rosemary, thyme, or oregano)
- Coarse sea salt or flaky salt for sprinkling

Optional Toppings:

- Sliced cherry tomatoes
- Pitted olives (black or green)
- Sliced red onions
- Fresh rosemary sprigs

Instructions:

1. In a large mixing bowl, combine bread flour and lukewarm water. Stir until all the flour is hydrated, cover the bowl, and let it rest for about 15-20 minutes. This step

is called the autolyse and helps improve the dough's extensibility.

2. After the autolyse, add the salt and active dry yeast to the dough. Mix until everything is well combined.

3. Add 30ml (2 tablespoons) of olive oil to the dough and knead it until the oil is fully incorporated. The dough will be sticky and wet.

4. Cover the bowl with a kitchen towel or plastic wrap and let the dough rise at room temperature for about 1 hour or until it has doubled in size.

5. Preheat your oven to 425°F (220°C) and generously grease a baking sheet with olive oil.

6. Gently deflate the risen dough and transfer it to the prepared baking sheet.

7. Stretch and press the dough into an even rectangle or oval shape, about 1-inch thick. If the dough resists, let it rest for a few minutes and try again.

8. Drizzle the remaining 30ml (2 tablespoons) of olive oil over the top of the dough, using your fingers to create dimples all over the surface.

9. Sprinkle the dried Italian herbs evenly over the dough, and add any optional toppings you desire, such as sliced cherry tomatoes, olives, red onions, or fresh rosemary.

10. Finish by sprinkling coarse sea salt or flaky salt over the entire surface.

11. Cover the dough with a kitchen towel and let it undergo the final proofing for about 30 minutes.

12. Once the focaccia has slightly puffed up, place it in the preheated oven and bake for 20-25 minutes or until the top is golden brown.

13. Remove the focaccia from the oven and transfer it to a wire rack to cool slightly.

14. Slice the focaccia into squares or wedges and serve warm or at room temperature.

Note: Focaccia is versatile, and you can customize it with various toppings, herbs, and seasonings according to your taste preferences.

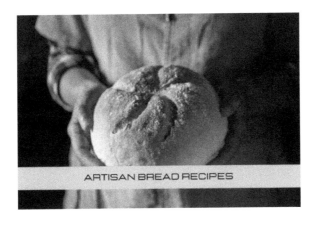

Rustic Olive Bread

Ingredients:

- 500g bread flour
- 400ml lukewarm water
- 10g salt
- 7g active dry yeast
- 2 tablespoons olive oil
- 1 cup pitted olives (black or green), chopped
- 2-3 tablespoons chopped fresh herbs (such as rosemary, thyme, or oregano)

Instructions:

1. In a large mixing bowl, combine bread flour and lukewarm water. Stir until all the flour is hydrated, cover the bowl, and let it rest for about 15-20 minutes. This step is called the autolyse and helps improve the dough's extensibility.
2. After the autolyse, add the salt and active dry yeast to the dough. Mix until everything is well combined.
3. Add the olive oil to the dough and knead it until the oil is fully incorporated. The dough will be slightly sticky.

4. Gently fold in the chopped olives and fresh herbs until they are evenly distributed throughout the dough.
5. Cover the bowl with a kitchen towel or plastic wrap and let the dough rise at room temperature for about 1 hour or until it has doubled in size.
6. Preheat your oven to 425°F (220°C) and generously grease a baking sheet or a baking stone with olive oil.
7. Gently deflate the risen dough and transfer it to the prepared baking sheet or baking stone.
8. Shape the dough into a round or oval loaf, about 1-inch thick.
9. Cover the dough with a kitchen towel and let it undergo the final proofing for about 30 minutes.
10. Once the bread has slightly puffed up, place it in the preheated oven and bake for 25-30 minutes or until the top is golden brown and the bottom sounds hollow when tapped.
11. Remove the Rustic Olive Bread from the oven and transfer it to a wire rack to cool slightly.
12. Slice the bread and serve warm or at room temperature, either on its own or paired with your favorite dishes.

Note:

You can use either black or green olives or a combination of both for a variety of flavors. Feel free to adjust the amount of olives and herbs based on your preference for a stronger or milder taste.

Enjoy the delightful combination of olives and fresh herbs in this homemade Rustic Olive Bread. Its wonderful aroma and savory taste will transport you to the Mediterranean with every bite. Whether enjoyed with a hearty Italian meal or as a stand-alone treat, this bread is sure to impress and satisfy.

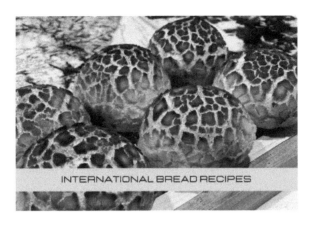

INTERNATIONAL BREAD RECIPES

Naan Bread (Indian)

Ingredients:

- 500g all-purpose flour
- 7g active dry yeast
- 1 teaspoon sugar
- 1 teaspoon salt
- 1/2 teaspoon baking powder
- 1/4 cup plain yogurt
- 1/4 cup milk
- 1/4 cup water
- 2 tablespoons vegetable oil (plus extra for brushing)
- 2-3 garlic cloves, minced (optional, for garlic naan)
- Fresh cilantro, chopped (optional, for garnish)

Instructions:

- In a small bowl, combine the milk and water. Warm the mixture to about 110°F (43°C). Add the sugar and active dry yeast to the warm milk-water mixture. Let it sit for about 5-10 minutes or until it becomes frothy.
- In a large mixing bowl, combine the all-purpose flour, salt, and baking powder.

- Make a well in the center of the dry ingredients and add the frothy yeast mixture, plain yogurt, and vegetable oil.

- Mix all the ingredients together to form a soft and slightly sticky dough.
- Transfer the dough to a floured surface and knead it for about 5-7 minutes or until it becomes smooth and elastic.
- Place the kneaded dough in a lightly oiled bowl, cover it with a damp kitchen towel or plastic wrap, and let it rise at room temperature for about 1 to 1.5 hours or until it doubles in size.
- Once the dough has risen, preheat a stovetop skillet or a grill over medium-high heat.
- Divide the dough into 6-8 equal-sized balls, depending on how big you want your naan.
- On a floured surface, roll out each dough ball into an oval or circular shape, about 1/4-inch thick.
- If making garlic naan, sprinkle minced garlic on one side of the rolled-out dough and press it lightly to adhere.
- Lightly brush one side of the rolled-out dough with water to help it stick to the cooking surface.
- Place the naan, water-brushed side down, on the preheated skillet or grill.
- Cook the naan for about 1-2 minutes on each side, or until it puffs up and develops golden brown spots.
- Once cooked, brush the top of the naan with a little vegetable oil for added flavor and softness.
- Repeat the process for the remaining dough balls.
- Garnish the naan with chopped fresh cilantro, if desired.

Note: You can also make stuffed naan by adding fillings such as cheese, minced meat, or vegetables before sealing the dough and rolling it out.

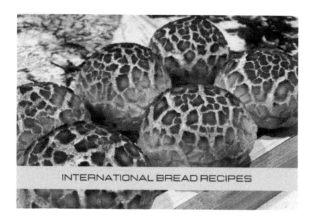

Pita Bread (Middle Eastern)

Ingredients:

- 500g all-purpose flour
- 7g active dry yeast
- 1 teaspoon sugar
- 1 teaspoon salt
- 1 cup lukewarm water
- 2 tablespoons olive oil (plus extra for brushing)

Instructions:

- In a small bowl, combine the lukewarm water, sugar, and active dry yeast. Let it sit for about 5-10 minutes or until it becomes frothy.
- In a large mixing bowl, combine the all-purpose flour and salt.
- Make a well in the center of the dry ingredients and pour in the frothy yeast mixture and olive oil.
- Mix all the ingredients together to form a dough.
- Transfer the dough to a floured surface and knead it for about 5-7 minutes or until it becomes smooth and elastic.

- Place the kneaded dough in a lightly oiled bowl, cover it with a damp kitchen towel or plastic wrap, and let it rise at room temperature for about 1 to 1.5 hours or until it doubles in size.
- Preheat your oven to 475°F (245°C) and place a baking stone or an inverted baking sheet on the middle rack.
- Once the dough has risen, gently deflate it and divide it into 8 equal-sized balls.
- On a floured surface, roll out each dough ball into a round shape, about 1/4-inch thick.
- Carefully transfer the rolled-out dough rounds onto a parchment-lined baking sheet.
- Let the dough rounds rest for about 10 minutes to relax the gluten.
- Place the baking sheet with the dough rounds onto the preheated baking stone or baking sheet in the oven.
- Bake the pita bread for about 4-5 minutes or until they puff up and turn golden brown.
- Once baked, remove the pita bread from the oven and brush them lightly with olive oil for added flavor and softness.
- Let the pita bread cool slightly on a wire rack.

Note: You can also cook the pita bread on a stovetop griddle or skillet over medium-high heat for about 2-3 minutes on each side until they puff up and get golden brown spots.If you prefer a thinner pita bread, you can roll out the dough rounds to a thinner thickness.

Enjoy the soft and versatile delight of this homemade Pita Bread, perfect for stuffing with your favorite Middle Eastern fillings or enjoyed as a side with dips and spreads. The warm, fresh-baked taste of these pocket breads will elevate your meals to a whole new level.

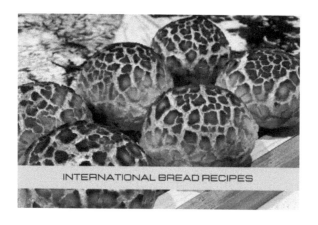

Swedish Rye Bread (Swedish)

Ingredients:

- 1 cup lukewarm water
- 1 package (7g) active dry yeast
- 1/4 cup molasses
- 2 tablespoons vegetable oil
- 1 teaspoon fennel seeds (optional, for added flavor)
- 1 teaspoon anise seeds (optional, for added flavor)
- 1 teaspoon caraway seeds (optional, for added flavor)
- 1/2 teaspoon ground cinnamon
- 1/2 teaspoon ground ginger
- 1/2 teaspoon salt
- 1 1/2 cups rye flour
- 1 1/2 cups all-purpose flour

Instructions:

1. In a large mixing bowl, combine lukewarm water and active dry yeast. Let it sit for about 5-10 minutes until it becomes frothy.
2. Add molasses, vegetable oil, fennel seeds, anise seeds, caraway seeds, ground cinnamon, ground ginger, and salt

to the yeast mixture. Stir until all the ingredients are well combined.

3. Gradually add rye flour and all-purpose flour to the wet mixture. Mix until a sticky dough forms.

4. Transfer the dough to a floured surface and knead it for about 5-7 minutes until it becomes smooth and elastic. You can use extra flour to prevent sticking, but keep in mind that the dough should remain slightly sticky.

5. Place the kneaded dough in a lightly oiled bowl, cover it with a damp kitchen towel or plastic wrap, and let it rise at room temperature for about 1 to 1.5 hours or until it doubles in size.

6. Preheat your oven to 375°F (190°C) and lightly grease a baking sheet or line it with parchment paper.

7. Once the dough has risen, gently deflate it and shape it into a round loaf or an oval shape.

8. Place the shaped dough on the prepared baking sheet.

9. Cover the dough with a kitchen towel and let it undergo the final proofing for about 30 minutes.

10. With a sharp knife or a razor blade, make a few shallow slashes on top of the dough for a decorative touch.

11. Bake the Swedish Rye Bread in the preheated oven for about 30-35 minutes or until it is golden brown and sounds hollow when tapped.

12. Once baked, remove the bread from the oven and let it cool on a wire rack.

Note:

The seeds and spices in this recipe are optional, but they add a distinct Swedish flavor to the bread. You can customize the spices according to your taste preferences. This bread is best enjoyed fresh, but it can be stored in an airtight container for a few days.

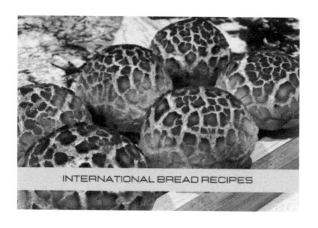

INTERNATIONAL BREAD RECIPES

Irish Soda Bread (Irish)

Ingredients:

- 4 cups all-purpose flour
- 1 teaspoon baking soda
- 1 teaspoon salt
- 1 3/4 cups buttermilk (or 1 3/4 cups milk + 1 tablespoon white vinegar or lemon juice)
- 2 tablespoons unsalted butter, melted

Optional Add-ins:

- 1/2 cup raisins or currants
- 1 tablespoon caraway seeds

Instructions:

1. Preheat your oven to 425°F (220°C). Lightly grease a baking sheet or line it with parchment paper.
2. In a large mixing bowl, whisk together the all-purpose flour, baking soda, and salt.
3. If you're adding raisins or currants and caraway seeds, stir them into the dry ingredients until evenly distributed.
4. In a separate bowl, mix the buttermilk and melted butter.

5. Make a well in the center of the dry ingredients and pour in the buttermilk-butter mixture.
6. Using a wooden spoon or your hands, gently mix the ingredients together until they form a soft and slightly sticky dough. Be careful not to overmix.
7. Turn the dough out onto a floured surface and shape it into a round loaf. The dough will be slightly sticky, so you can lightly flour your hands to help with shaping.
8. Transfer the shaped dough to the prepared baking sheet.
9. Using a sharp knife, make a shallow "X" on top of the dough, about 1/2 inch deep. This helps the bread bake evenly and allows the center to cook properly.
10. Bake the Irish Soda Bread in the preheated oven for about 35-40 minutes or until it is golden brown and sounds hollow when tapped on the bottom.
11. Once baked, remove the bread from the oven and let it cool on a wire rack.
12. Enjoy the Irish Soda Bread warm or at room temperature, sliced and served with butter, jam, or your favorite spreads.

Note:

Traditional Irish Soda Bread does not contain sugar, eggs, or other sweeteners. It's meant to be a simple and hearty bread that pairs well with savory dishes. If you don't have buttermilk, you can make a buttermilk substitute by adding 1 tablespoon of white vinegar or lemon juice to 1 3/4 cups of milk and letting it sit for a few minutes until it curdles.

Indulge in the rustic and wholesome delight of this homemade Irish Soda Bread, perfect for enjoying the taste of Ireland in your own kitchen. Whether served as part of a St. Patrick's Day feast or as an everyday treat, this traditional bread is sure to be a hit.

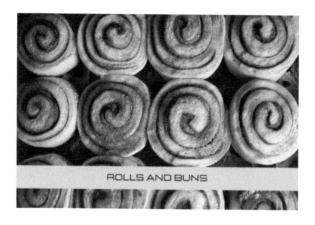

Dinner Rolls

Ingredients:

- 4 cups all-purpose flour
- 1/4 cup granulated sugar
- 1 teaspoon salt
- 1 package (7g) active dry yeast
- 1 cup warm milk (about 110°F/43°C)
- 1/4 cup unsalted butter, melted
- 1 large egg, at room temperature
- Extra melted butter for brushing (optional)

Instructions:

1. In a large mixing bowl, combine 3 cups of all-purpose flour, granulated sugar, salt, and active dry yeast.
2. In a separate bowl, whisk together warm milk, melted butter, and the egg until well combined.
3. Pour the wet ingredients into the dry ingredients, and mix until a soft dough forms.
4. Gradually add the remaining 1 cup of all-purpose flour, a little at a time, until the dough is smooth and no longer

sticks to the bowl or your hands. You may not need to use the entire cup of flour.

5. Transfer the dough to a lightly floured surface and knead it for about 5-7 minutes until it becomes smooth and elastic.
6. Place the kneaded dough in a lightly oiled bowl, cover it with a damp kitchen towel or plastic wrap, and let it rise at room temperature for about 1 to 1.5 hours or until it doubles in size.
7. Once the dough has risen, gently deflate it and divide it into 12 equal-sized balls.
8. Shape each ball into a smooth round roll and place them on a lightly greased baking pan, leaving a little space between each roll.
9. Cover the rolls with a kitchen towel and let them undergo the final proofing for about 30 minutes.
10. Preheat your oven to 375°F (190°C).
11. If desired, lightly brush the top of the rolls with melted butter for a golden finish.
12. Bake the Dinner Rolls in the preheated oven for about 15-20 minutes or until they turn golden brown.
13. Once baked, remove the rolls from the oven and let them cool slightly on a wire rack.
14. Serve the warm and fluffy Dinner Rolls alongside your favorite meals or enjoy them with butter or jam.

Note:

You can shape the dinner rolls into different shapes, such as crescent or square, by gently pulling and shaping the dough accordingly. If you prefer a richer flavor, you can use whole milk or add a little honey to the dough for a touch of sweetness.

Indulge in the soft and delectable delight of these homemade Dinner Rolls, perfect for elevating your dinner table with the goodness of freshly baked bread.

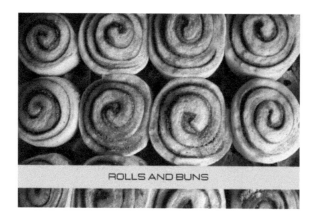

ROLLS AND BUNS

Cinnamon Rolls

Ingredients For the dough:

- 4 cups all-purpose flour
- 1/3 cup granulated sugar
- 1 teaspoon salt
- 1 package (7g) active dry yeast
- 3/4 cup warm milk (about 110°F/43°C)
- 1/4 cup unsalted butter, melted
- 1/4 cup warm water
- 2 large eggs, at room temperature

For the filling:

- 1/2 cup unsalted butter, softened
- 1 cup packed brown sugar
- 2 tablespoons ground cinnamon

For the cream cheese frosting:

- 1/4 cup unsalted butter, softened
- 4 ounces cream cheese, softened
- 1 teaspoon vanilla extract
- 1 1/2 cups powdered sugar

Instructions For the dough:

1. In a large mixing bowl, combine 3 cups of all-purpose flour, granulated sugar, salt, and active dry yeast.
2. In a separate bowl, whisk together warm milk, melted butter, warm water, and eggs until well combined.
3. Pour the wet ingredients into the dry ingredients, and mix until a soft dough forms.
4. Gradually add the remaining 1 cup of all-purpose flour, a little at a time, until the dough is smooth and slightly sticky.
5. Transfer the dough to a lightly floured surface and knead it for about 5-7 minutes until it becomes smooth and elastic.
6. Place the kneaded dough in a lightly oiled bowl, cover it with a damp kitchen towel or plastic wrap, and let it rise at room temperature for about 1 to 1.5 hours or until it doubles in size.

For the filling: In a small bowl, mix together softened butter, brown sugar, and ground cinnamon until well combined.

Assembly and baking:

1. Preheat your oven to 375°F (190°C). Grease a baking dish or line it with parchment paper.
2. Once the dough has risen, gently deflate it and roll it out into a large rectangle, about 16x12 inches.
3. Spread the cinnamon-sugar filling evenly over the rolled-out dough, leaving a small border around the edges.
4. Starting from one long side, tightly roll up the dough into a log.
5. Using a sharp knife or dental floss, cut the log into 12 equal-sized rolls.
6. Place the rolls in the prepared baking dish, leaving a little space between each roll.
7. Cover the rolls with a kitchen towel and let them undergo the final proofing for about 30 minutes.

8. Bake the Cinnamon Rolls in the preheated oven for about 20-25 minutes or until they turn golden brown.

For the cream cheese frosting:

1. In a mixing bowl, beat together softened butter, cream cheese, and vanilla extract until smooth.
2. Gradually add powdered sugar to the cream cheese mixture, and continue beating until the frosting is smooth and creamy.

Assembly:

1. Once the rolls are baked, remove them from the oven and let them cool slightly in the baking dish.
2. Spread the cream cheese frosting over the warm rolls.
3. Serve the Cinnamon Rolls warm and enjoy this sweet, gooey, and delectable treat!

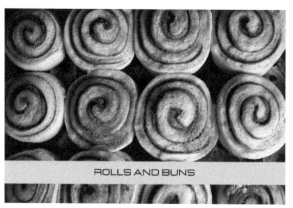

ROLLS AND BUNS

Garlic Knots

Ingredients For the dough:

- 4 cups all-purpose flour
- 1 package (7g) active dry yeast
- 1 1/2 cups warm water (about 110°F/43°C)
- 2 tablespoons olive oil
- 1 tablespoon granulated sugar

- 1 teaspoon salt

For the garlic butter:

- 1/2 cup unsalted butter, melted
- 4 cloves garlic, minced
- 1/4 cup fresh parsley, chopped
- 1/2 teaspoon salt
- 1/4 teaspoon black pepper
- Pinch of red pepper flakes (optional, for a bit of heat)

Instructions For the dough:

1. In a large mixing bowl, combine warm water, granulated sugar, and active dry yeast. Let it sit for about 5-10 minutes until it becomes frothy.
2. Add olive oil and salt to the yeast mixture.
3. Gradually add all-purpose flour to the wet mixture. Mix until a soft dough forms.
4. Transfer the dough to a floured surface and knead it for about 5-7 minutes until it becomes smooth and elastic.
5. Place the kneaded dough in a lightly oiled bowl, cover it with a damp kitchen towel or plastic wrap, and let it rise at room temperature for about 1 to 1.5 hours or until it doubles in size.

For the garlic butter:

In a small bowl, mix together melted butter, minced garlic, chopped parsley, salt, black pepper, and red pepper flakes (if using). Set aside.

Assembly and baking:

1. Preheat your oven to 375°F (190°C). Grease a baking dish or line it with parchment paper.
2. Once the dough has risen, gently deflate it and divide it into 20 equal-sized pieces.
3. Roll each piece into a rope about 8 inches long.
4. Tie each rope into a knot and tuck the ends underneath.

5. Place the garlic knots in the prepared baking dish, leaving a little space between each knot.
6. Cover the knots with a kitchen towel and let them undergo the final proofing for about 20-30 minutes.
7. After the final proofing, brush the garlic butter mixture over each garlic knot, making sure to coat them evenly.
8. Bake the Garlic Knots in the preheated oven for about 15-20 minutes or until they turn golden brown.
9. Once baked, remove the knots from the oven and let them cool slightly in the baking dish.

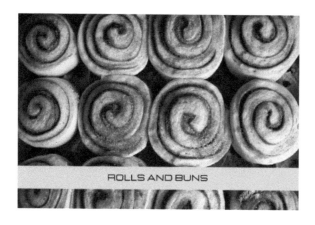

ROLLS AND BUNS

Pretzel Buns

Ingredients For the dough:

- 4 cups all-purpose flour
- 1 package (7g) active dry yeast
- 1 1/4 cups warm water (about 110°F/43°C)
- 2 tablespoons unsalted butter, melted
- 2 tablespoons granulated sugar
- 1 teaspoon salt

For the pretzel bath:

- 10 cups water
- 2/3 cup baking soda

For the topping Coarse sea salt or pretzel salt

Instructions For the dough:

1. In a large mixing bowl, combine warm water, granulated sugar, and active dry yeast. Let it sit for about 5-10 minutes until it becomes frothy.
2. Add melted butter and salt to the yeast mixture.
3. Gradually add all-purpose flour to the wet mixture. Mix until a soft dough forms.
4. Transfer the dough to a floured surface and knead it for about 5-7 minutes until it becomes smooth and elastic.
5. Place the kneaded dough in a lightly oiled bowl, cover it with a damp kitchen towel or plastic wrap, and let it rise at room temperature for about 1 to 1.5 hours or until it doubles in size.

For the pretzel bath:

1. Preheat your oven to 425°F (220°C). Line a baking sheet with parchment paper.
2. In a large pot, bring 10 cups of water to a boil. Once boiling, add the baking soda (be cautious, as it may cause the water to bubble up).

Assembly and baking:

1. Once the dough has risen, gently deflate it and divide it into 8 equal-sized pieces.
2. Roll each piece into a smooth ball and then slightly flatten it into a disc shape.
3. Dip each dough disc into the boiling water bath with baking soda for about 30 seconds, flipping it halfway through.
4. Using a slotted spoon, remove the dough discs from the water bath and place them on the prepared baking sheet.
5. Sprinkle coarse sea salt or pretzel salt over the top of each bun.
6. Using a sharp knife or a razor blade, make a shallow "X" on top of each bun for a decorative touch.

7. Bake the Pretzel Buns in the preheated oven for about 12-15 minutes or until they turn golden brown.
8. Once baked, remove the buns from the oven and let them cool slightly on a wire rack.

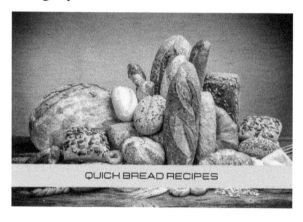

QUICH BREAD RECIPES

Zucchini Bread

Ingredients:

- 2 cups all-purpose flour
- 1 teaspoon baking powder
- 1/2 teaspoon baking soda
- 1/2 teaspoon salt
- 1 teaspoon ground cinnamon
- 1/2 teaspoon ground nutmeg
- 1/4 teaspoon ground cloves
- 2 large eggs, at room temperature
- 1/2 cup vegetable oil or melted butter
- 1 cup granulated sugar
- 1/2 cup packed brown sugar
- 1 teaspoon vanilla extract
- 1 1/2 cups grated zucchini (about 1 medium zucchini)
- 1/2 cup chopped walnuts or pecans (optional)
- 1/2 cup raisins or chocolate chips (optional)

Instructions:

1. Preheat your oven to 350°F (175°C). Grease and flour a 9x5-inch loaf pan or line it with parchment paper.
2. In a large mixing bowl, whisk together the all-purpose flour, baking powder, baking soda, salt, ground cinnamon, ground nutmeg, and ground cloves.
3. In a separate bowl, beat the eggs lightly. Add vegetable oil (or melted butter), granulated sugar, brown sugar, and vanilla extract. Mix until well combined.
4. Add the grated zucchini to the wet ingredients and stir until evenly distributed.
5. Gradually add the dry ingredients to the wet ingredients and mix until just combined. Be careful not to overmix the batter.
6. If using, fold in the chopped walnuts or pecans and the raisins or chocolate chips.
7. Pour the batter into the prepared loaf pan, spreading it out evenly.
8. Bake the Zucchini Bread in the preheated oven for about 50-60 minutes or until a toothpick inserted into the center comes out clean.
9. Once baked, remove the bread from the oven and let it cool in the pan for about 10 minutes.
10. Transfer the bread to a wire rack to cool completely before slicing.

Note: You can also make Zucchini Bread muffins by dividing the batter among muffin cups and baking for about 18-22 minutes.

You can adjust the amount of spices and add other flavors like grated orange zest or ground ginger for variation.

Enjoy the moist and flavorful delight of this homemade Zucchini Bread, perfect for enjoying the goodness of zucchini in a sweet and delicious form. Whether served as a breakfast treat or as an afternoon snack, this zucchini bread is sure to be a favorite with friends and family.

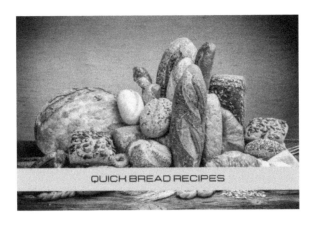

QUICH BREAD RECIPES

Banana Nut Bread

Ingredients:

- 2 cups all-purpose flour
- 1 teaspoon baking soda
- 1/2 teaspoon baking powder
- 1/2 teaspoon salt
- 1 teaspoon ground cinnamon
- 1/2 cup unsalted butter, softened
- 3/4 cup granulated sugar
- 2 large eggs, at room temperature
- 3 ripe bananas, mashed (about 1 cup)
- 1 teaspoon vanilla extract
- 1/2 cup chopped walnuts or pecans

Instructions:

1. Preheat your oven to 350°F (175°C). Grease and flour a 9x5-inch loaf pan or line it with parchment paper.
2. In a large mixing bowl, whisk together the all-purpose flour, baking soda, baking powder, salt, and ground cinnamon.
3. In a separate bowl, cream the softened butter and granulated sugar until light and fluffy.

4. Add the eggs one at a time, beating well after each addition.
5. Stir in the mashed bananas and vanilla extract until well combined.
6. Gradually add the dry ingredients to the wet ingredients, mixing until just combined. Be careful not to overmix the batter.
7. Fold in the chopped walnuts or pecans, reserving a few for sprinkling on top.
8. Pour the batter into the prepared loaf pan, spreading it out evenly.
9. Sprinkle the remaining chopped nuts over the top of the batter.
10. Bake the Banana Nut Bread in the preheated oven for about 50-60 minutes or until a toothpick inserted into the center comes out clean.
11. Once baked, remove the bread from the oven and let it cool in the pan for about 10 minutes.
12. Transfer the bread to a wire rack to cool completely before slicing.

Note: For added sweetness and texture, you can also add 1/2 cup of raisins or chocolate chips to the batter. Make sure to use ripe bananas with brown spots for the best flavor in the bread.

Enjoy the moist and nutty delight of this homemade Banana Nut Bread, perfect for breakfast or as a satisfying snack. Whether served warm with a dollop of butter or enjoyed with a cup of coffee, this classic banana nut bread is sure to bring comfort and joy to your taste buds.

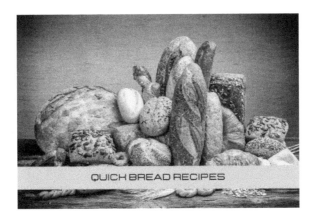

Lemon Blueberry Bread

Ingredients:

- 2 cups all-purpose flour
- 1 teaspoon baking powder
- 1/2 teaspoon baking soda
- 1/4 teaspoon salt
- 1 cup granulated sugar
- Zest of 1 large lemon
- 1/2 cup unsalted butter, softened
- 2 large eggs, at room temperature
- 1 teaspoon vanilla extract
- 1/2 cup fresh lemon juice
- 1/2 cup buttermilk (or 1/2 cup milk + 1 tablespoon white vinegar or lemon juice)
- 1 1/2 cups fresh blueberries, rinsed and dried

For the lemon glaze (optional):

- 1 cup powdered sugar
- 2-3 tablespoons fresh lemon juice

Instructions:

1. Preheat your oven to 350°F (175°C). Grease and flour a 9x5-inch loaf pan or line it with parchment paper.
2. In a large mixing bowl, whisk together the all-purpose flour, baking powder, baking soda, and salt.
3. In a separate bowl, rub the lemon zest into the granulated sugar until fragrant and well combined.
4. Add the softened butter to the lemon-sugar mixture and cream together until light and fluffy.
5. Beat in the eggs one at a time, followed by the vanilla extract.
6. Mix in the fresh lemon juice and buttermilk until well combined.
7. Gradually add the dry ingredients to the wet ingredients, mixing until just combined. Be careful not to overmix the batter.
8. Gently fold in the fresh blueberries until evenly distributed throughout the batter.
9. Pour the batter into the prepared loaf pan, spreading it out evenly.
10. Bake the Lemon Blueberry Bread in the preheated oven for about 55-65 minutes or until a toothpick inserted into the center comes out clean.
11. Once baked, remove the bread from the oven and let it cool in the pan for about 10 minutes.

For the lemon glaze (optional):

1. In a small bowl, whisk together powdered sugar and fresh lemon juice until you achieve a smooth glaze consistency.
2. Drizzle the lemon glaze over the cooled Lemon Blueberry Bread.

Note: You can use either fresh or frozen blueberries for this recipe. If using frozen, do not thaw them before adding to the batter. If you don't have buttermilk, you can make a buttermilk substitute by adding 1 tablespoon of white vinegar or lemon juice to 1/2 cup of milk and letting it sit for a few minutes until it curdles.

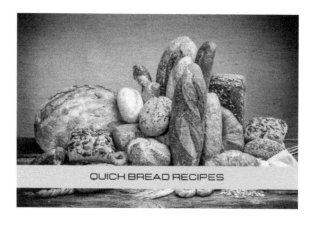

QUICK BREAD RECIPES

Chocolate Marble Bread

Ingredients:

- 2 cups all-purpose flour
- 1 teaspoon baking powder
- 1/2 teaspoon baking soda
- 1/4 teaspoon salt
- 1 cup granulated sugar
- 1/2 cup unsalted butter, softened
- 2 large eggs, at room temperature
- 1 teaspoon vanilla extract
- 1 cup buttermilk (or 1 cup milk + 1 tablespoon white vinegar or lemon juice)
- 1/4 cup unsweetened cocoa powder
- 1/4 cup hot water
- 1/2 cup chocolate chips (optional)

Instructions:

1. Preheat your oven to 350°F (175°C). Grease and flour a 9x5-inch loaf pan or line it with parchment paper.
2. In a large mixing bowl, whisk together the all-purpose flour, baking powder, baking soda, and salt.

3. In a separate bowl, cream together the softened butter and granulated sugar until light and fluffy.
4. Beat in the eggs one at a time, followed by the vanilla extract.
5. Mix in the buttermilk until well combined.
6. Gradually add the dry ingredients to the wet ingredients, mixing until just combined. Be careful not to overmix the batter.
7. In a small bowl, mix the unsweetened cocoa powder with hot water until smooth to create the chocolate batter.
8. Divide the vanilla batter in half. Stir the chocolate batter into one half of the vanilla batter until fully incorporated.
9. Spoon alternate dollops of vanilla and chocolate batter into the prepared loaf pan.
10. Using a knife or skewer, gently swirl the batters together to create a marbled pattern.
11. If using chocolate chips, sprinkle them over the top of the batter.
12. Bake the Chocolate Marble Bread in the preheated oven for about 55-65 minutes or until a toothpick inserted into the center comes out clean.
13. Once baked, remove the bread from the oven and let it cool in the pan for about 10 minutes.
14. Transfer the bread to a wire rack to cool completely before slicing.

Note: You can customize the chocolate marble bread by adding chopped nuts or a swirl of peanut butter or Nutella for extra flavor and texture. If you don't have buttermilk, you can make a buttermilk substitute by adding 1 tablespoon of white vinegar or lemon juice to 1 cup of milk and letting it sit for a few minutes until it curdles.

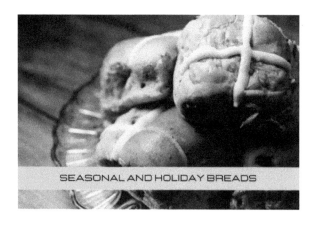

Hot Cross Buns (Easter)

Ingredients For the buns:

- 4 cups all-purpose flour
- 1/2 cup granulated sugar
- 1 package (7g) active dry yeast
- 1 teaspoon ground cinnamon
- 1/4 teaspoon ground nutmeg
- 1/4 teaspoon ground cloves
- 1/2 teaspoon salt
- 1 cup warm milk (about 110°F/43°C)
- 1/4 cup unsalted butter, melted
- 1/4 cup warm water
- 1 large egg, at room temperature
- 1/2 cup currants or raisins

For the cross topping: 1/2 cup all-purpose flour - 1/4 cup water

For the glaze: 1/4 cup granulated sugar - 1/4 cup water

Instructions For the buns:

1. In a large mixing bowl, whisk together 3 cups of all-purpose flour, granulated sugar, active dry yeast, ground cinnamon, ground nutmeg, ground cloves, and salt.

2. In a separate bowl, mix warm milk, melted butter, warm water, and the egg until well combined.
3. Make a well in the center of the dry ingredients and pour in the milk-butter mixture.
4. Stir the mixture until it forms a soft dough.
5. Turn the dough out onto a floured surface and knead it for about 5-7 minutes until it becomes smooth and elastic.
6. Place the kneaded dough in a lightly oiled bowl, cover it with a damp kitchen towel or plastic wrap, and let it rise at room temperature for about 1 to 1.5 hours or until it doubles in size.
7. Once the dough has risen, gently deflate it and knead in the currants or raisins until evenly distributed.
8. Divide the dough into 12 equal-sized pieces and shape each piece into a smooth round ball.
9. Place the balls of dough on a greased or parchment-lined baking sheet, leaving a little space between each bun.

For the cross topping:

1. In a small bowl, mix together 1/2 cup all-purpose flour and 1/4 cup water until you achieve a thick paste.
2. Transfer the paste into a piping bag or a small plastic sandwich bag with the corner snipped off.
3. Pipe a cross on top of each bun using the flour paste.

Baking:

1. Preheat your oven to 375°F (190°C).
2. Let the buns undergo the final proofing for about 20-30 minutes while the oven preheats.
3. Once the buns have risen, bake them in the preheated oven for about 15-20 minutes or until they turn golden brown.

For the glaze:

1. In a small saucepan, mix together 1/4 cup granulated sugar and 1/4 cup water.

2. Heat the mixture over low heat until the sugar dissolves and a syrup forms.

Assembly: As soon as the buns come out of the oven, brush the glaze over the top of each bun while they are still warm. Let the Hot Cross Buns cool slightly on a wire rack before serving.

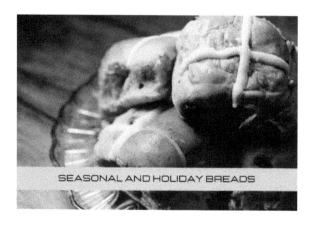

SEASONAL AND HOLIDAY BREADS

King Cake (Mardi Gras)

Ingredients For the cake dough:

- 4 cups all-purpose flour
- 1/2 cup granulated sugar
- 1 package (7g) active dry yeast
- 1 teaspoon salt
- 1/2 cup whole milk
- 1/4 cup water
- 1/2 cup unsalted butter, softened
- 4 large eggs, at room temperature
- 1 teaspoon vanilla extract
- 1 teaspoon grated lemon zest (optional)

For the filling:

- 1/2 cup packed brown sugar
- 2 teaspoons ground cinnamon

- 1/4 cup unsalted butter, softened

For the glaze:

- 2 cups powdered sugar
- 3 tablespoons whole milk
- 1/2 teaspoon vanilla extract
- Colored sugar or icing (in purple, green, and gold)

Instructions For the cake dough:

1. In a large mixing bowl, whisk together 3 cups of all-purpose flour, granulated sugar, active dry yeast, and salt.
2. In a small saucepan, heat the milk, water, and softened butter over low heat until the butter melts and the mixture is warm but not boiling.
3. Add the warm milk mixture to the dry ingredients and mix until well combined.
4. Add the eggs, one at a time, beating well after each addition.
5. Stir in the vanilla extract and grated lemon zest (if using).
6. Gradually add the remaining 1 cup of all-purpose flour, a little at a time, until the dough is soft and slightly sticky.
7. Turn the dough out onto a floured surface and knead it for about 5-7 minutes until it becomes smooth and elastic.
8. Place the kneaded dough in a lightly oiled bowl, cover it with a damp kitchen towel or plastic wrap, and let it rise at room temperature for about 1 to 1.5 hours or until it doubles in size.

For the filling:

1. In a small bowl, mix together the packed brown sugar, ground cinnamon, and softened butter until you achieve a smooth paste.
2. Assembly and baking:
3. Preheat your oven to 375°F (190°C). Grease a large baking sheet or line it with parchment paper.
4. Once the dough has risen, gently deflate it and roll it out into a large rectangle, about 24x12 inches.
5. Spread the filling evenly over the rolled-out dough, leaving a small border around the edges.

6. Starting from one long side, tightly roll up the dough into a log.
7. Shape the log into a circle and pinch the ends together to seal it, forming a ring.
8. Place the ring on the prepared baking sheet and let it undergo the final proofing for about 20-30 minutes.
9. Bake the King Cake in the preheated oven for about 25-30 minutes or until it turns golden brown.

For the glaze: In a small bowl, whisk together the powdered sugar, whole milk, and vanilla extract until you achieve a smooth glaze.

Decoration: Once the King Cake has cooled, drizzle the glaze over the top of the cake. Sprinkle colored sugar or icing in purple, green, and gold over the glaze in alternating sections to create the traditional Mardi Gras colors.

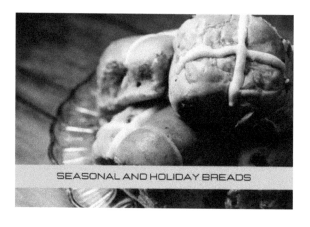

SEASONAL AND HOLIDAY BREADS

Irish Soda Bread with Raisins (St. Patrick's Day)

Ingredients:

- 4 cups all-purpose flour
- 1/4 cup granulated sugar
- 1 teaspoon baking soda
- 1 teaspoon baking powder

- 1/2 teaspoon salt
- 1/2 cup (1 stick) unsalted butter, cold and cubed
- 1 1/2 cups buttermilk (or 1 1/2 cups milk + 1 tablespoon white vinegar or lemon juice)
- 1 cup raisins

Instructions:

1. Preheat your oven to 375°F (190°C). Grease a baking sheet or line it with parchment paper.
2. In a large mixing bowl, whisk together the all-purpose flour, granulated sugar, baking soda, baking powder, and salt.
3. Add the cold cubed butter to the dry ingredients. Using a pastry cutter or your fingertips, work the butter into the flour mixture until it resembles coarse crumbs.
4. Stir in the raisins until evenly distributed.
5. Make a well in the center of the mixture and pour in the buttermilk.
6. Stir the mixture with a wooden spoon or your hands until it comes together into a soft, slightly sticky dough. Be careful not to overmix.
7. Turn the dough out onto a floured surface and gently knead it for a minute to bring it together.
8. Shape the dough into a round loaf and place it on the prepared baking sheet.
9. Use a sharp knife to make a shallow "X" on top of the dough, about 1/2 inch deep. This helps the bread cook evenly.
10. Bake the Irish Soda Bread in the preheated oven for about 40-45 minutes or until it turns golden brown and sounds hollow when tapped on the bottom.
11. Once baked, remove the bread from the oven and let it cool on a wire rack before slicing.

Note: If you don't have buttermilk, you can make a buttermilk substitute by adding 1 tablespoon of white vinegar or lemon juice to 1 1/2 cups of milk and letting it sit for a few minutes until it curdles. You can customize this Irish Soda Bread by adding other dried fruits, such as currants or dried cranberries, for variation.

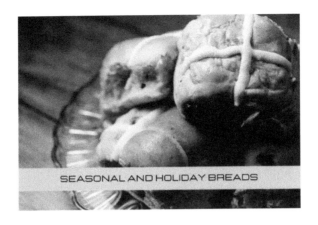

Spiced Pumpkin Bread (Thanksgiving)

Ingredients:

- 2 cups all-purpose flour
- 1 teaspoon baking soda
- 1/2 teaspoon baking powder
- 1/2 teaspoon salt
- 1 teaspoon ground cinnamon
- 1/2 teaspoon ground nutmeg
- 1/4 teaspoon ground cloves
- 1 1/2 cups granulated sugar
- 1/2 cup vegetable oil or melted butter
- 2 large eggs, at room temperature
- 1 teaspoon vanilla extract
- 1 3/4 cups canned pumpkin puree (not pumpkin pie filling)
- 1/2 cup water

Instructions:

1. Preheat your oven to 350°F (175°C). Grease and flour a 9x5-inch loaf pan or line it with parchment paper.

91

2. In a large mixing bowl, whisk together the all-purpose flour, baking soda, baking powder, salt, ground cinnamon, ground nutmeg, and ground cloves.
3. In a separate bowl, whisk together the granulated sugar, vegetable oil or melted butter, eggs, and vanilla extract until well combined.
4. Stir in the canned pumpkin puree until well incorporated.
5. Gradually add the dry ingredients to the wet ingredients, alternating with the water, mixing until just combined. Be careful not to overmix the batter.
6. Pour the batter into the prepared loaf pan, spreading it out evenly.
7. Bake the Spiced Pumpkin Bread in the preheated oven for about 60-70 minutes or until a toothpick inserted into the center comes out clean.
8. Once baked, remove the bread from the oven and let it cool in the pan for about 10 minutes.
9. Transfer the bread to a wire rack to cool completely before slicing.

Note: You can add chopped nuts (such as walnuts or pecans) or raisins to the batter for added texture and flavor if desired. If you prefer a stronger spice flavor, you can adjust the amount of cinnamon, nutmeg, and cloves to your taste.

Enjoy the warm and comforting delight of this homemade Spiced Pumpkin Bread, perfect for celebrating Thanksgiving or anytime you crave the flavors of fall. Whether served with a smear of butter, cream cheese, or as a complement to a Thanksgiving feast, this spiced pumpkin bread is sure to be a favorite with family and friends.

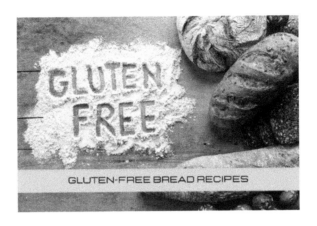

GLUTEN-FREE BREAD RECIPES

Gluten-Free White Bread

Ingredients:

- 2 1/2 cups gluten-free all-purpose flour blend (make sure it contains xanthan gum or add 1 teaspoon separately)
- 1 1/2 teaspoons active dry yeast
- 1 1/2 teaspoons sugar
- 1 teaspoon salt
- 1 cup warm water (about 110°F/43°C)
- 2 tablespoons olive oil or melted butter
- 3 large eggs, at room temperature
- 1 teaspoon apple cider vinegar

Instructions:

1. In a small bowl, mix warm water, sugar, and active dry yeast. Let it sit for about 5-10 minutes until it becomes frothy.
2. In a large mixing bowl, whisk together the gluten-free all-purpose flour blend and salt.
3. In a separate bowl, beat the eggs, then add the olive oil (or melted butter) and apple cider vinegar. Mix until well combined.

93

4. Pour the yeast mixture into the egg-oil mixture and stir until fully incorporated.
5. Gradually add the wet ingredients to the dry ingredients, mixing until you get a smooth and thick batter. The batter should be more like a cake batter than a traditional bread dough.
6. Grease a 9x5-inch loaf pan and pour the batter into it, smoothing the top with a spatula.
7. Cover the loaf pan with a damp kitchen towel or plastic wrap and let the bread rise in a warm place for about 1 to 1.5 hours or until it reaches the top of the pan.
8. Preheat your oven to 375°F (190°C) while the bread is rising.
9. Once the bread has risen, bake it in the preheated oven for about 40-45 minutes or until the top is golden brown and a toothpick inserted into the center comes out clean.
10. Once baked, remove the bread from the oven and let it cool in the pan for about 10 minutes.
11. Transfer the bread to a wire rack to cool completely before slicing.

Note: Store any leftovers in an airtight container at room temperature for a few days or freeze individual slices for longer storage.

Enjoy the soft and gluten-free goodness of this homemade Gluten-Free White Bread, perfect for sandwiches, toasts, or any occasion. Whether served with your favorite spreads or used to make delicious gluten-free sandwiches, this bread is sure to satisfy anyone following a gluten-free lifestyle.

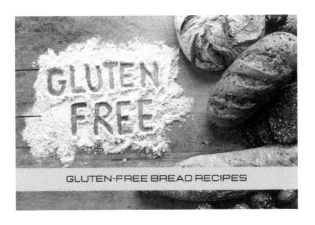

GLUTEN-FREE BREAD RECIPES

Gluten-Free Cinnamon Raisin Bread

Ingredients:

- 2 cups gluten-free all-purpose flour blend (make sure it contains xanthan gum or add 1 teaspoon separately)
- 1 teaspoon baking powder
- 1/2 teaspoon baking soda
- 1/2 teaspoon salt
- 1 teaspoon ground cinnamon
- 1/2 cup granulated sugar
- 1/2 cup milk (dairy or plant-based)
- 1/4 cup vegetable oil or melted butter
- 2 large eggs, at room temperature
- 1 teaspoon vanilla extract
- 1 cup raisins

Instructions:

1. Preheat your oven to 350°F (175°C). Grease and flour a 9x5-inch loaf pan or line it with parchment paper.
2. In a large mixing bowl, whisk together the gluten-free all-purpose flour blend, baking powder, baking soda, salt, ground cinnamon, and granulated sugar.

3. In a separate bowl, whisk together the milk, vegetable oil (or melted butter), eggs, and vanilla extract until well combined.
4. Pour the wet ingredients into the dry ingredients and mix until you get a smooth batter.
5. Stir in the raisins until evenly distributed throughout the batter.
6. Pour the batter into the prepared loaf pan, spreading it out evenly.
7. Bake the Gluten-Free Cinnamon Raisin Bread in the preheated oven for about 45-55 minutes or until a toothpick inserted into the center comes out clean.
8. Once baked, remove the bread from the oven and let it cool in the pan for about 10 minutes.
9. Transfer the bread to a wire rack to cool completely before slicing.

Note: Store any leftovers in an airtight container at room temperature for a few days or freeze individual slices for longer storage. You can also add chopped nuts, such as walnuts or pecans, for added texture and flavor if desired.

Enjoy the wonderful aroma and taste of this homemade Gluten-Free Cinnamon Raisin Bread, perfect for breakfast or as a special treat. Whether served toasted with butter or cream cheese or enjoyed as is, this gluten-free version of the classic cinnamon raisin bread is sure to be a favorite with those who follow a gluten-free lifestyle.

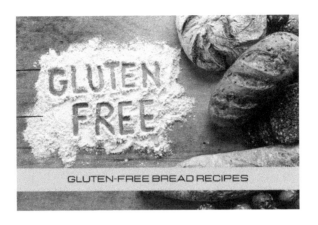

GLUTEN-FREE BREAD RECIPES

Gluten-Free Rosemary and Garlic Bread

Ingredients:

- 2 cups gluten-free all-purpose flour blend (make sure it contains xanthan gum or add 1 teaspoon separately)
- 1 teaspoon baking powder
- 1/2 teaspoon baking soda
- 1/2 teaspoon salt
- 2 tablespoons fresh rosemary, finely chopped
- 3 cloves garlic, minced
- 1/2 cup milk (dairy or plant-based)
- 1/4 cup vegetable oil or melted butter
- 2 large eggs, at room temperature
- 1 teaspoon apple cider vinegar

Instructions:

1. Preheat your oven to 350°F (175°C). Grease and flour a 9x5-inch loaf pan or line it with parchment paper.
2. In a large mixing bowl, whisk together the gluten-free all-purpose flour blend, baking powder, baking soda, salt, finely chopped rosemary, and minced garlic.

3. In a separate bowl, whisk together the milk, vegetable oil (or melted butter), eggs, and apple cider vinegar until well combined.
4. Pour the wet ingredients into the dry ingredients and mix until you get a smooth batter.
5. Transfer the batter into the prepared loaf pan, spreading it out evenly.
6. If desired, you can brush the top of the batter with a little extra oil or melted butter and sprinkle some additional chopped rosemary and minced garlic on top for added flavor and presentation.
7. Bake the Gluten-Free Rosemary and Garlic Bread in the preheated oven for about 45-50 minutes or until a toothpick inserted into the center comes out clean.
8. Once baked, remove the bread from the oven and let it cool in the pan for about 10 minutes.
9. Transfer the bread to a wire rack to cool completely before slicing.

Note: Store any leftovers in an airtight container at room temperature for a few days or freeze individual slices for longer storage. If you prefer a stronger garlic flavor, you can adjust the amount of minced garlic to your taste.

Enjoy the savory and aromatic delight of this homemade Gluten-Free Rosemary and Garlic Bread, perfect for accompanying soups, salads, or enjoyed on its own as a flavorful snack. Whether served warm or at room temperature, this gluten-free bread is sure to be a hit with family and friends.

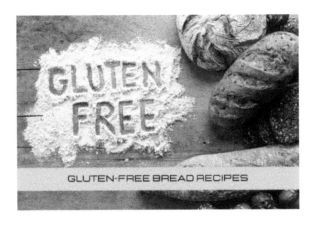

GLUTEN-FREE BREAD RECIPES

Gluten-Free Banana Bread

Ingredients:

- 2 cups gluten-free all-purpose flour blend (make sure it contains xanthan gum or add 1 teaspoon separately)
- 1 teaspoon baking powder
- 1/2 teaspoon baking soda
- 1/2 teaspoon salt
- 1 teaspoon ground cinnamon
- 1/2 cup granulated sugar
- 1/4 cup vegetable oil or melted butter
- 2 large eggs, at room temperature
- 4 ripe bananas, mashed
- 1 teaspoon vanilla extract
- 1/2 cup chopped nuts (such as walnuts or pecans), optional

Instructions:

1. Preheat your oven to 350°F (175°C). Grease and flour a 9x5-inch loaf pan or line it with parchment paper.
2. In a large mixing bowl, whisk together the gluten-free all-purpose flour blend, baking powder, baking soda, salt, ground cinnamon, and granulated sugar.

3. In a separate bowl, whisk together the vegetable oil (or melted butter), eggs, mashed bananas, and vanilla extract until well combined.
4. Pour the wet ingredients into the dry ingredients and mix until you get a smooth batter.
5. If desired, fold in the chopped nuts for added texture and flavor.
6. Pour the batter into the prepared loaf pan, spreading it out evenly.
7. If you like, you can add sliced bananas on top for an extra visual touch.
8. Bake the Gluten-Free Banana Bread in the preheated oven for about 55-65 minutes or until a toothpick inserted into the center comes out clean.
9. Once baked, remove the bread from the oven and let it cool in the pan for about 10 minutes.
10. Transfer the bread to a wire rack to cool completely before slicing.

Note: Store any leftovers in an airtight container at room temperature for a few days or freeze individual slices for longer storage. You can customize this gluten-free banana bread by adding chocolate chips, dried fruits, or coconut flakes if desired.

Enjoy the moist and flavorful delight of this homemade Gluten-Free Banana Bread, perfect for any occasion. Whether served warm with a smear of butter or as a comforting treat on its own, this gluten-free version of banana bread is sure to be a hit with everyone.

Brean Machine Cookbook

@2023 Alessia Sofia Ferrari

BREAD MACHINE
RECIPES

The Bread Machine Cookbook

40 Recipes for Every Occasion

Second Edition

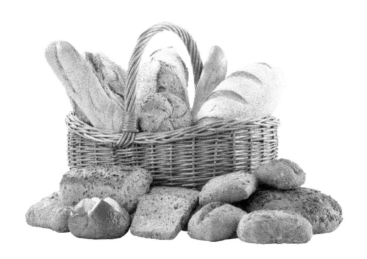

Alessia Sofia Ferrari

Bread Machine Cookbook

@2023 Alessia Sofia Ferrari

INTRODUCTION

The enchanting scent of freshly baked bread fills the air, evoking nostalgic memories of home and warmth. Within the pages of "Freshly Baked Perfection: 45 Irresistible Recipes for Your Bread Machine," we welcome you to embark on a delightful journey into the realm of bread machines. Discover the joy of effortlessly baking delicious homemade bread, making every moment in the kitchen a rewarding and magical experience.

The Bread Machine Revolution

No more laborious kneading or waiting for dough to rise; the days of uncertainty in achieving the perfect loaf are gone. The bread machine has revolutionized the art of baking, bringing the delights of homemade bread to kitchens all around the globe. These compact wonders eliminate the guesswork from bread making, automating the entire process from mixing to baking. Now, you have the freedom to focus on life's finer aspects while savoring the joys of freshly baked bread at home.

Why Choose a Bread Machine?

The answer lies in simplicity – convenience and consistency. With a bread machine as your trusty companion, creating a variety of breads for any occasion becomes effortless. Whether it's a hearty breakfast, a wholesome family meal, or a delightful afternoon snack, your bread machine has you covered. From classic white loaves to specialty artisanal creations, the possibilities are limitless.

The Joy of Baking at Your Fingertips

No longer do you need to rush to the bakery or settle for store-bought loaves with unknown ingredients. "Freshly Baked Perfection" puts the power of baking into your hands, allowing you to craft delectable, freshly baked bread whenever your heart desires. Each recipe has been thoughtfully curated to cater to diverse tastes, ensuring there's something for everyone to savor and enjoy.

Our Promise to You

In "Freshly Baked Perfection," our mission is to demystify the art of bread making and empower bakers of all levels with confidence. Whether you're an experienced pro or a novice, our step-by-step instructions will walk you through the process, ensuring consistently outstanding results.

Embrace the Joy of Homemade Bread

Baking bread carries a sense of nostalgia and tradition, connecting us to our heritage and allowing us to show love and care to those we share it with. Embark on a culinary adventure with us, as the heartwarming scent of freshly baked bread fills your kitchen with love, comfort, and joy.

Prepare to experience the satisfaction of crafting your own bread masterpieces, tailored to your preferences and dietary needs. Your bread machine opens the gateway to a world of flavors, textures, and creativity that will delight your taste buds and those of your loved ones. So, let's preheat those ovens, gather our ingredients, and dive into the delightful world of bread machine baking.

Benefits of using a bread machine for baking

Using a bread machine for baking brings numerous advantages, making it an indispensable kitchen appliance for bread enthusiasts. Let's explore some of the key benefits:

1. Time-Saving Convenience: Traditional bread-making involves multiple time-consuming steps like kneading, rising, and baking. With a bread machine, you simply add the ingredients, select the settings, and let the machine handle the rest. This frees up your time for other activities while still enjoying freshly baked bread.

2. Foolproof Baking: Bread machines take the guesswork out of baking. With precise settings for kneading, rising, and baking, you can achieve consistent and reliable results every time, even if you're a novice baker.

3. Customizable Recipes: Bread machines allow you to customize recipes to suit your preferences. Whether you want to adjust sweetness, add grains, seeds, or make gluten-free alternatives, the machine empowers you to experiment and create personalized bread variations.

4. Freshness and Flavor: The aroma and taste of freshly baked bread are incomparable. With a bread machine, you can wake up or come home to the comforting fragrance of warm bread. Enjoying bread at its freshest enhances its flavor and texture, a delight for your taste buds.

5. Healthier Ingredients: Baking bread at home gives you control over ingredients. Choose high-quality, organic, and locally sourced options, eliminating artificial additives or preservatives found in store-bought bread. This lets you create healthier and more wholesome bread for your family.

6. Cost-Effective: Over time, baking bread at home with a machine can be cost-effective, saving money on store-bought bread, especially if you consume bread regularly.

7. Versatility: Bread machines are not limited to basic recipes. Many models offer settings for making dough for various treats like pizza, pasta, and cinnamon rolls. This versatility expands your baking options and encourages culinary exploration.

8. Reduced Energy Consumption: Bread machines are designed to be energy-efficient, using less energy compared to traditional ovens, making them an eco-friendly choice for the environmentally conscious.

Ideal for Beginners and Busy Individuals: For newcomers to bread-making or those with busy schedules, a bread machine is a game-changer. It eliminates the need for hands-on work and monitoring, making baking stress-free and accessible.

General tips for successful bread machine baking

To ensure successful bread machine baking and achieve delicious, perfectly baked loaves, keep these general tips in mind:

1. Precise Measurements: Accurate measuring of ingredients is vital for successful bread machine baking. Use appropriate measuring tools for dry and liquid ingredients, and select the right type of flour as specified in the recipe.

2. Follow the Recipe: Even with a bread machine, carefully follow the recipe instructions. Different bread machine models may have specific requirements for ingredient order and settings.

3. Fresh Ingredients: Use fresh and high-quality ingredients for the best results. Check the expiration date of yeast and leavening agents, as expired ingredients can affect the bread's rise and flavor.

4. Adjust Liquid and Flour Ratios: Depending on humidity and altitude, you may need to adjust the amount of liquid or flour in the recipe. The dough should form a smooth ball without being too sticky or dry.

5. Avoid Overmixing: Let the bread machine handle the mixing and kneading process. Avoid opening the lid during these phases to prevent overmixing, which can lead to tough bread.

6. Add Mix-ins at the Right Time: If your recipe includes mix-ins, add them at the appropriate time during the baking cycle. Many bread machines have an alert for adding mix-ins.

7. Check Dough Consistency: Peek inside the bread machine during the kneading phase to ensure the dough is the right consistency. Adjust with additional liquid or flour as needed.

8. Grease the Bread Pan: Lightly grease the bread pan to prevent sticking and make it easier to remove the finished loaf.

9. Mindful of Yeast Placement: When using delayed start settings, ensure the yeast doesn't touch the liquid prematurely. Place the yeast on top of the flour to keep it dry until the machine starts.

10. Room Temperature Ingredients: Use room temperature eggs, milk, and other refrigerated ingredients for proper yeast activation and even baking.

11. Select the Right Settings: Choose the appropriate setting for the type of bread you're making, such as white bread, whole wheat, or sweet bread.

12. Promptly Remove the Bread: Once baking is complete, remove the bread promptly to prevent it from becoming soggy due to residual heat.

13. Let It Cool: Allow the bread to cool on a wire rack for at least 20-30 minutes before slicing to avoid a gummy texture.

By following these tips, you'll master the art of bread machine baking and enjoy a delightful array of freshly baked bread from the comfort of your home.

Overview of essential ingredients and equipment

Essential Equipment:

- Bread Machine: A reliable bread machine is the heart of your bread-making journey. Choose a model with appropriate size and features to suit your baking needs.
- Bread Pan: The removable pan inside the bread machine where you'll place the ingredients and where the bread will bake.
- Measuring Tools: Accurate measuring cups and spoons for dry and liquid ingredients are essential for precise measurements.
- Spatula: Use a spatula to scrape down the sides of the bread pan and ensure all ingredients are properly mixed.
- Cooling Rack: After baking, transfer the bread to a cooling rack to prevent the bottom from becoming soggy.

With these ingredients and equipment at your disposal, you're well-equipped to embark on your bread machine baking adventure. Follow recipes carefully, experiment with different ingredients, and enjoy the delightful experience of freshly baked bread right in your own kitchen!

Equipment:

- Bread Machine: The star of the show! Choose a reliable bread machine with settings that suit your baking needs. Some machines have advanced features like gluten-free settings, crust color options, and delay start timers.
- Measuring Cups and Spoons: Accurate measurements are crucial for successful baking. Invest in a set of dry and liquid measuring cups and spoons.

- Mixing Bowl: While the bread machine handles the mixing and kneading, you might need a mixing bowl for some recipes that require additional hand mixing.
- Bread Pans: Most bread machines come with a removable bread pan. Ensure it's clean and properly greased before adding the ingredients.
- Cooling Rack: After baking, allow the bread to cool on a wire cooling rack to avoid condensation and maintain the crust's texture.
- Oven Mitts or Kitchen Towels: Bread machine pans and freshly baked bread can be hot. Protect your hands with oven mitts or kitchen towels when handling them.
- Bread Knife or Slicer: For perfectly even slices, use a bread knife or slicer when the loaf has cooled.

With these essential ingredients and equipment, you're ready to dive into the world of bread machine baking. Enjoy creating a variety of delightful breads to satisfy your cravings and impress your loved ones. Happy baking!

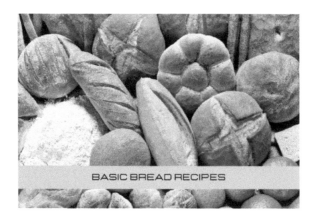

BASIC BREAD RECIPES

Rye Bread

Ingredients:

- 1 cup warm water (about 110°F / 45°C)
- 2 1/4 teaspoons active dry yeast
- 1/4 cup honey or molasses
- 1 tablespoon vegetable oil
- 1 teaspoon salt
- 1 cup rye flour
- 2 1/2 cups bread flour (all-purpose flour can also be used)
- 1 tablespoon caraway seeds (optional, for added flavor and texture)

Instructions:

1. In a large mixing bowl, combine the warm water and yeast. Let it sit for 5 minutes until the yeast becomes frothy.
2. Stir in the honey (or molasses) and vegetable oil into the yeast mixture.
3. Add the salt, rye flour, and 2 cups of bread flour (reserve the remaining 1/2 cup for later) to the wet ingredients. If using caraway seeds, add them at this stage as well.

4. Mix the ingredients with a wooden spoon until a rough dough forms.
5. Turn the dough out onto a lightly floured surface and knead for about 8-10 minutes, adding more bread flour as needed, until the dough becomes smooth, elastic, and slightly tacky to the touch.
6. Shape the dough into a ball and place it in a greased bowl. Cover the bowl with a clean kitchen towel or plastic wrap.
7. Allow the dough to rise in a warm, draft-free place for about 1 to 1.5 hours, or until it doubles in size.
8. Preheat your oven to 375°F (190°C). If you have a baking stone or pizza stone, place it in the oven while preheating.
9. Punch down the risen dough and shape it into a loaf. You can use a loaf pan or shape it free-form on a baking sheet or parchment paper.
10. Cover the shaped loaf and let it rise for another 30-45 minutes, or until it rises slightly above the edges of the pan or holds its shape if free-form.
11. Optional: Score the top of the loaf with a sharp knife to create a decorative pattern.
12. Place the risen loaf in the preheated oven (on the baking stone, if using) and bake for 30-35 minutes, or until the crust is deep golden brown and the loaf sounds hollow when tapped on the bottom.
13. Remove the bread from the oven and let it cool on a wire rack before slicing.

Enjoy your freshly baked homemade Rye Bread! This bread pairs wonderfully with soups, sandwiches, or simply toasted with butter or your favorite spread. Store any leftovers in an airtight container to keep it fresh for a few days.

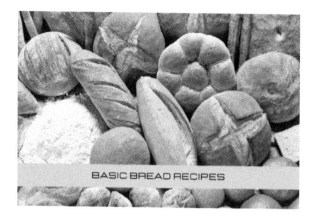

French Baguette

Ingredients:

- 2 1/4 teaspoons (1 packet) active dry yeast
- 1 1/2 cups warm water (about 110°F / 45°C)
- 1 tablespoon granulated sugar
- 1 tablespoon olive oil
- 1 1/2 teaspoons salt
- 3 1/2 cups all-purpose flour
- Cornmeal (for dusting)

Instructions:

1. In a large mixing bowl, combine the warm water and sugar. Sprinkle the yeast over the water and let it sit for about 5 minutes until the yeast becomes frothy.
2. Stir in the olive oil and salt into the yeast mixture.
3. Gradually add the all-purpose flour to the wet ingredients, stirring with a wooden spoon until a shaggy dough forms.
4. Turn the dough out onto a lightly floured surface and knead for about 8-10 minutes, until the dough becomes smooth, elastic, and slightly tacky to the touch.

116

5. Shape the dough into a ball and place it in a lightly greased bowl. Cover the bowl with a clean kitchen towel or plastic wrap.
6. Allow the dough to rise in a warm, draft-free place for about 1 to 1.5 hours, or until it doubles in size.
7. Preheat your oven to 450°F (230°C). If you have a baking stone or pizza stone, place it in the oven while preheating.
8. Punch down the risen dough and turn it out onto a lightly floured surface.
9. Divide the dough into two equal portions and shape each portion into a long, thin baguette shape. You can use your hands or gently roll the dough into a long log.
10. Place the shaped baguettes on a baking sheet lined with parchment paper or a silicone baking mat. Alternatively, you can place them on a baguette pan, if available.
11. Dust the parchment paper or pan with cornmeal to prevent sticking.
12. Optional: Using a sharp knife or a razor blade, make 3-4 diagonal slashes on the top of each baguette for a classic baguette appearance.
13. Cover the baguettes with a clean kitchen towel and let them rise for another 20-30 minutes.
14. Transfer the risen baguettes (still on the parchment paper, if using) onto the preheated baking stone or directly onto the oven rack.
15. Bake the baguettes for 20-25 minutes, or until they develop a golden brown crust.
16. Remove the baguettes from the oven and let them cool on a wire rack before slicing.

Enjoy your freshly baked Classic French Baguette! These baguettes are perfect for serving with soups, stews, or using as the base for delicious sandwiches. To keep the baguettes fresh, store them in a paper bag or loosely wrapped in a clean kitchen towel.

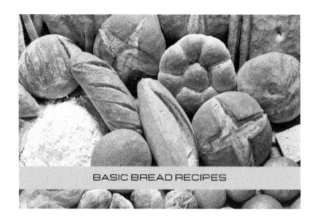

Brioche Bread

Ingredients:

- 1/4 cup warm water (about 110°F / 45°C)
- 2 1/4 teaspoons (1 packet) active dry yeast
- 1/3 cup granulated sugar
- 4 cups all-purpose flour
- 1 teaspoon salt
- 5 large eggs, at room temperature
- 1/2 cup unsalted butter, softened
- 1 egg yolk (for egg wash)
- 1 tablespoon milk (for egg wash)

Instructions:

1. In a small bowl, combine the warm water and 1 tablespoon of sugar. Sprinkle the yeast over the water and let it sit for about 5 minutes until the yeast becomes frothy.
2. In a large mixing bowl, whisk together the flour, remaining sugar, and salt.
3. Add the frothy yeast mixture and 4 of the eggs to the dry ingredients. Mix the dough with a wooden spoon until it starts to come together.
4. Transfer the dough to a floured surface and knead for about 10-12 minutes, until the dough becomes smooth and elastic.

118

5. Gradually add the softened butter, one tablespoon at a time, kneading well after each addition. Continue kneading until the butter is fully incorporated into the dough and the dough becomes soft and silky.
6. Shape the dough into a ball and place it in a lightly greased bowl. Cover the bowl with a clean kitchen towel or plastic wrap.
7. Allow the dough to rise in a warm, draft-free place for about 2 to 2.5 hours, or until it doubles in size.
8. Punch down the risen dough and turn it out onto a floured surface.

9. Divide the dough into two equal portions. You can shape each portion into a loaf for a classic brioche bread or into smaller portions for individual brioches.
10. Place the shaped dough into greased loaf pans or brioche molds.
11. In a small bowl, whisk together the egg yolk and milk to create the egg wash.
12. Brush the egg wash over the top of the shaped dough to give the brioche a beautiful golden color when baked.
13. Cover the pans or molds with a clean kitchen towel and let the dough rise for another 1 to 1.5 hours, or until it rises slightly above the edges of the pans or molds.
14. Preheat your oven to 375°F (190°C).
15. Once the dough has risen, place the pans or molds in the preheated oven.
16. Bake the brioche for 25-30 minutes for individual brioches or 35-40 minutes for a larger loaf, or until the top turns golden brown and the bread sounds hollow when tapped on the bottom.
17. Remove the brioche from the oven and let it cool in the pans or molds for a few minutes before transferring to a wire rack to cool completely.

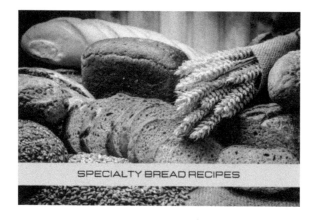

SPECIALTY BREAD RECIPES

Sunflower Seed Bread

Ingredients:

- 1 3/4 cups all-purpose flour
- 1 teaspoon baking soda
- 1/2 teaspoon baking powder
- 1/2 teaspoon salt
- 1 teaspoon ground cinnamon
- 1/2 teaspoon ground ginger
- 1/4 teaspoon ground nutmeg
- 1/4 teaspoon ground cloves
- 1 cup pumpkin puree
- 1/2 cup vegetable oil
- 1 cup granulated sugar
- 1/2 cup brown sugar
- 2 large eggs, at room temperature
- 1/3 cup water
- 1 teaspoon vanilla extract

Instructions:

1. Preheat your oven to 350°F (175°C). Grease a 9x5-inch loaf pan and set it aside.
2. In a medium mixing bowl, whisk together the flour, baking soda, baking powder, salt, ground cinnamon, ground ginger, ground nutmeg, and ground cloves. Set the dry ingredients aside.
3. In a large mixing bowl, whisk together the pumpkin puree, vegetable oil, granulated sugar, and brown sugar until well combined.
4. Add the eggs, one at a time, to the pumpkin mixture, whisking well after each addition.
5. Stir in the water and vanilla extract until the wet ingredients are fully combined.
6. Gradually add the dry ingredients to the wet ingredients, mixing with a wooden spoon or spatula until just combined. Be careful not to overmix.
7. Pour the batter into the greased loaf pan, spreading it evenly.
8. Optional: For a decorative touch, sprinkle some extra brown sugar or pumpkin seeds on top of the batter.
9. Bake the pumpkin spice bread in the preheated oven for 55-60 minutes or until a toothpick inserted into the center comes out clean.
10. Remove the bread from the oven and let it cool in the pan for about 10 minutes.
11. Carefully transfer the bread from the pan to a wire rack to cool completely.
12. Once cooled, slice and enjoy your delicious Homemade Pumpkin Spice Bread! This bread is perfect for autumn mornings, afternoon snacks, or as a delightful dessert. Store any leftovers in an airtight container to keep them fresh.

Note: Feel free to add chopped nuts, raisins, or chocolate chips to the batter for additional texture and flavor if desired.

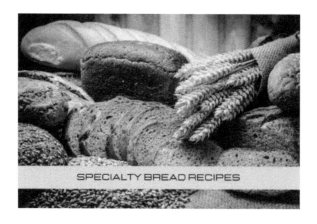

SPECIALTY BREAD RECIPES

Chocolate Chip Banana Bread

Ingredients:

- 2 cups all-purpose flour
- 1 teaspoon baking powder
- 1/2 teaspoon baking soda
- 1/2 teaspoon salt
- 1 teaspoon ground cinnamon
- 1/2 cup unsalted butter, softened
- 3/4 cup granulated sugar
- 2 large eggs, at room temperature
- 4 ripe bananas, mashed
- 1 teaspoon vanilla extract
- 1/3 cup sour cream or plain yogurt
- 1 cup semi-sweet chocolate chips

Instructions:

- Preheat your oven to 350°F (175°C). Grease a 9x5-inch loaf pan and set it aside.
- In a medium mixing bowl, whisk together the flour, baking powder, baking soda, salt, and ground cinnamon. Set the dry ingredients aside.

- In a large mixing bowl, cream the softened butter and granulated sugar together using a hand mixer or stand mixer until light and fluffy.
- Add the eggs one at a time, beating well after each addition.
- Mix in the mashed bananas and vanilla extract until well combined.
- Gradually add the dry ingredients to the wet ingredients, alternating with the sour cream or plain yogurt, in three batches. Start and end with the dry ingredients. Mix until just combined after each addition.
- Gently fold in the chocolate chips into the banana bread batter.
- Pour the batter into the greased loaf pan, spreading it evenly.
- Optional: For an extra touch, sprinkle a few more chocolate chips on top of the batter.
- Bake the banana bread in the preheated oven for 60-70 minutes or until a toothpick inserted into the center comes out with a few moist crumbs (not wet batter).
- If the top of the bread starts to brown too quickly during baking, you can cover it with foil halfway through to prevent over-browning.
- Remove the banana bread from the oven and let it cool in the pan for about 10 minutes.
- Carefully transfer the bread from the pan to a wire rack to cool completely.
- Slice and indulge in your Irresistible Chocolate Chip Banana Bread! This delightful treat is perfect for breakfast, snack time, or as a sweet treat any time of the day. Store any leftovers in an airtight container to keep them fresh.

Note: You can customize this recipe by adding chopped nuts or using different types of chocolate chips (milk chocolate, dark chocolate, or a combination)..

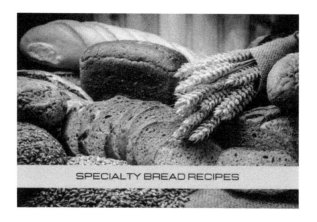

SPECIALTY BREAD RECIPES

Gluten-Free Bread

Ingredients:

- 2 cups gluten-free all-purpose flour blend (store-bought or homemade)
- 1 teaspoon xanthan gum (if not included in the flour blend)
- 1 teaspoon baking powder
- 1/2 teaspoon baking soda
- 1/2 teaspoon salt
- 1 tablespoon active dry yeast
- 1 1/4 cups warm water (about 110°F / 45°C)
- 2 tablespoons honey or maple syrup
- 2 large eggs, at room temperature
- 2 tablespoons olive oil or melted butter
- 1 teaspoon apple cider vinegar

Instructions:

1. Preheat your oven to 375°F (190°C). Grease a 9x5-inch loaf pan or line it with parchment paper. Set it aside.
2. In a large mixing bowl, whisk together the gluten-free all-purpose flour blend, xanthan gum (if needed), baking powder, baking soda, and salt.

3. In a small bowl, combine the warm water and honey (or maple syrup). Sprinkle the active dry yeast over the water and let it sit for about 5 minutes until the yeast becomes frothy.
4. In another small bowl, whisk together the eggs, olive oil (or melted butter), and apple cider vinegar.
5. Add the yeast mixture and the egg mixture to the dry ingredients. Mix with a wooden spoon or spatula until well combined and smooth. The batter will be thick and sticky.
6. Transfer the batter to the greased loaf pan, smoothing the top with a spatula or wet fingers.
7. Cover the pan with a clean kitchen towel or plastic wrap and let the bread rise in a warm, draft-free place for about 60-75 minutes, or until it rises slightly above the edges of the pan.
8. Preheat the oven to 375°F (190°C) if not already preheated.
9. Bake the gluten-free bread in the preheated oven for 35-40 minutes or until the top is golden brown and the bread sounds hollow when tapped on the bottom.
10. Remove the bread from the oven and let it cool in the pan for about 10 minutes.
11. Carefully transfer the bread from the pan to a wire rack to cool completely.
12. Once cooled, slice and savor your Delicious Gluten-Free Bread! This bread is perfect for those with gluten sensitivities or those looking for a tasty gluten-free alternative. Store any leftovers in an airtight container to keep them fresh.

Note: Gluten-free flours can vary, so feel free to experiment with different gluten-free all-purpose flour blends or mixtures. Adding seeds or nuts to the batter can also enhance the texture and flavor of the bread.

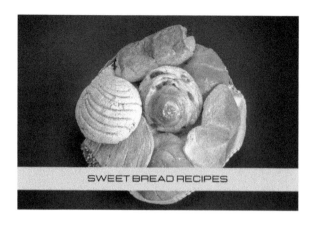

SWEET BREAD RECIPES

Apricot Almond Bread

Ingredients:

- 1 1/2 cups all-purpose flour
- 1 teaspoon baking powder
- 1/2 teaspoon baking soda
- 1/2 teaspoon salt
- 1/2 cup unsalted butter, softened
- 3/4 cup granulated sugar
- 2 large eggs, at room temperature
- 1 teaspoon almond extract
- 1/2 cup plain yogurt or sour cream
- 1/4 cup milk
- 1/2 cup dried apricots, chopped
- 1/2 cup almonds, chopped (plus extra for topping)
- 1 tablespoon apricot jam (optional, for glazing)

Instructions:

1. Preheat your oven to 350°F (175°C). Grease a 9x5-inch loaf pan and set it aside.
2. In a medium mixing bowl, whisk together the flour, baking powder, baking soda, and salt. Set the dry ingredients aside.

3. In a large mixing bowl, cream the softened butter and granulated sugar together using a hand mixer or stand mixer until light and fluffy.
4. Add the eggs one at a time, beating well after each addition.
5. Mix in the almond extract, plain yogurt (or sour cream), and milk until well combined.
6. Gradually add the dry ingredients to the wet ingredients, mixing with a wooden spoon or spatula until just combined.
7. Gently fold in the chopped dried apricots and chopped almonds into the batter.
8. Pour the batter into the greased loaf pan, spreading it evenly.
9. Optional: Sprinkle some extra chopped almonds on top of the batter for added texture and decoration.
10. Bake the apricot almond bread in the preheated oven for 45-55 minutes or until a toothpick inserted into the center comes out clean.
11. If the top of the bread starts to brown too quickly during baking, you can cover it with foil halfway through to prevent over-browning.
12. While the bread is still warm, you can brush the top with apricot jam for a glossy glaze (optional).
13. Remove the bread from the oven and let it cool in the pan for about 10 minutes.
14. Carefully transfer the bread from the pan to a wire rack to cool completely.
15. Slice and enjoy your Heavenly Apricot Almond Bread! This delightful bread is perfect for breakfast, brunch, or as a delightful treat with a cup of tea or coffee. Store any leftovers in an airtight container to keep them fresh.

Note: You can also use almond flour or almond meal to add a more pronounced almond flavor and texture to the bread. If you prefer a sweeter bread, you can increase the sugar to 1 cup or add a sprinkle of powdered sugar on top before serving.

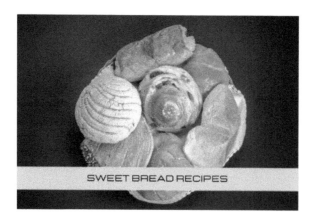

SWEET BREAD RECIPES

Blueberry Streusel Bread

Ingredients For the Streusel Topping:

- 1/4 cup all-purpose flour
- 1/4 cup granulated sugar
- 2 tablespoons unsalted butter, cold and cubed
- 1/2 teaspoon ground cinnamon

For the Bread:

- 2 cups all-purpose flour
- 1 teaspoon baking powder
- 1/2 teaspoon baking soda
- 1/2 teaspoon salt
- 1/2 cup unsalted butter, softened
- 3/4 cup granulated sugar
- 2 large eggs, at room temperature
- 1 teaspoon vanilla extract
- 1/2 cup plain yogurt or sour cream
- 1/4 cup milk
- 1 1/2 cups fresh or frozen blueberries

Instructions:

1. Preheat your oven to 350°F (175°C). Grease a 9x5-inch loaf pan and set it aside.

2. To make the streusel topping, in a small bowl, mix together the all-purpose flour, granulated sugar, cold cubed butter, and ground cinnamon. Use your fingers or a fork to blend the ingredients until the mixture resembles coarse crumbs. Set the streusel topping aside.

3. In a medium mixing bowl, whisk together the flour, baking powder, baking soda, and salt. Set the dry ingredients aside.
4. In a large mixing bowl, cream the softened butter and granulated sugar together using a hand mixer or stand mixer until light and fluffy.
5. Add the eggs one at a time, beating well after each addition.
6. Mix in the vanilla extract, plain yogurt (or sour cream), and milk until well combined.
7. Gradually add the dry ingredients to the wet ingredients, mixing with a wooden spoon or spatula until just combined.
8. Gently fold in the blueberries into the batter, being careful not to crush them.
9. Pour the batter into the greased loaf pan, spreading it evenly.
10. Sprinkle the streusel topping over the batter, covering it evenly.
11. Bake the blueberry streusel bread in the prcheated oven for 55-65 minutes or until a toothpick inserted into the center comes out clean.
12. If the top of the bread starts to brown too quickly during baking, you can cover it with foil halfway through to prevent over-browning.
13. Remove the bread from the oven and let it cool in the pan for about 10 minutes.
14. Carefully transfer the bread from the pan to a wire rack to cool completely.
15. Slice and enjoy your Delectable Blueberry Streusel Bread! This moist and flavorful bread is perfect for breakfast, brunch, or as a delightful snack any time of the day. Store any leftovers in an airtight container to keep them fresh.

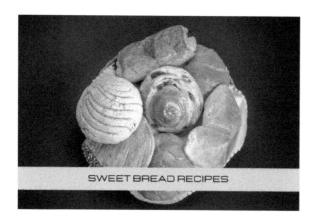

SWEET BREAD RECIPES

Apple Cinnamon Bread

Ingredients:

- 2 cups all-purpose flour
- 1 teaspoon baking powder
- 1/2 teaspoon baking soda
- 1/4 teaspoon salt
- 1/2 cup unsalted butter, softened
- 3/4 cup granulated sugar
- 2 large eggs, at room temperature
- 1 teaspoon vanilla extract
- 1 cup buttermilk (or 1 cup milk mixed with 1 tablespoon white vinegar or lemon juice)
- 1/2 cup Nutella (or any chocolate hazelnut spread)

Instructions:

1. Preheat your oven to 350°F (175°C). Grease a 9x5-inch loaf pan and set it aside.
2. In a medium mixing bowl, whisk together the flour, baking powder, baking soda, and salt. Set the dry ingredients aside.
3. In a large mixing bowl, cream the softened butter and granulated sugar together using a hand mixer or stand mixer until light and fluffy.
4. Add the eggs one at a time, beating well after each addition.

5. Mix in the vanilla extract until well combined.
6. Gradually add the dry ingredients to the wet ingredients, alternating with the buttermilk, in three batches. Start and end with the dry ingredients. Mix until just combined after each addition.
7. Pour half of the batter into the greased loaf pan, spreading it evenly.
8. Spoon dollops of Nutella over the batter in the pan, then use a knife or a skewer to gently swirl the Nutella through the batter.
9. Pour the remaining half of the batter over the Nutella layer, spreading it evenly.
10. Add more dollops of Nutella on top of the second layer of batter, and swirl it again with a knife or skewer.
11. Optional: You can sprinkle a few chocolate chips on top for an extra touch of chocolate goodness.
12. Bake the Nutella swirl bread in the preheated oven for 55-65 minutes or until a toothpick inserted into the center comes out clean.
13. If the top of the bread starts to brown too quickly during baking, you can cover it with foil halfway through to prevent over-browning.
14. Remove the bread from the oven and let it cool in the pan for about 10 minutes.
15. Carefully transfer the bread from the pan to a wire rack to cool completely.
16. Slice and indulge in your Irresistible Nutella Swirl Bread! This delightful treat is perfect for breakfast, snack time, or as a sweet dessert. Store any leftovers in an airtight container to keep them fresh.

Note: The Nutella swirls can be adjusted to your liking. You can add more or less Nutella depending on how chocolatey you want the bread to be.

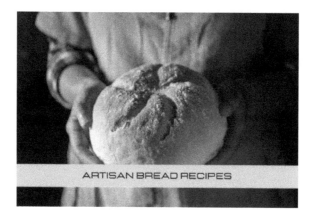

Pesto and Parmesan Bread

Ingredients:

- 2 cups all-purpose flour
- 1 teaspoon baking powder
- 1/2 teaspoon baking soda
- 1/2 teaspoon salt
- 1/2 cup unsalted butter, softened
- 1/2 cup grated Parmesan cheese
- 2 tablespoons store-bought or homemade pesto sauce
- 2 large eggs, at room temperature
- 1 cup buttermilk (or 1 cup milk mixed with 1 tablespoon white vinegar or lemon juice)
- 1/4 cup chopped fresh basil (optional, for added flavor and garnish)

Instructions:

1. Preheat your oven to 350°F (175°C). Grease a 9x5-inch loaf pan and set it aside.
2. In a medium mixing bowl, whisk together the flour, baking powder, baking soda, and salt. Set the dry ingredients aside.
3. In a large mixing bowl, cream the softened butter and grated Parmesan cheese together using a hand mixer or stand mixer until well combined.

4. Mix in the pesto sauce until evenly distributed in the butter and cheese mixture.
5. Add the eggs one at a time, beating well after each addition.
6. Gradually add the dry ingredients to the wet ingredients, alternating with the buttermilk, in three batches. Start and end with the dry ingredients. Mix until just combined after each addition.
7. Gently fold in the chopped fresh basil (if using) into the batter.
8. Pour the batter into the greased loaf pan, spreading it evenly.
9. Optional: You can sprinkle some additional grated Parmesan cheese on top for a golden and cheesy crust.
10. Bake the pesto and Parmesan bread in the preheated oven for 45-55 minutes or until a toothpick inserted into the center comes out clean.
11. If the top of the bread starts to brown too quickly during baking, you can cover it with foil halfway through to prevent over-browning.
12. Remove the bread from the oven and let it cool in the pan for about 10 minutes.
13. Carefully transfer the bread from the pan to a wire rack to cool completely.
14. Slice and savor your Savory Pesto and Parmesan Bread! This bread is a delightful addition to any meal, whether served as a side with pasta, soup, or as a delicious snack on its own. Store any leftovers in an airtight container to keep them fresh.

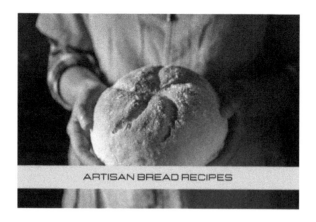

Cranberry Walnut Artisan Bread

Ingredients:

- 3 cups all-purpose flour
- 1 teaspoon active dry yeast
- 1 1/2 teaspoons salt
- 1 1/2 cups warm water (around 110°F or 45°C)
- 1/2 cup dried cranberries
- 1/2 cup chopped walnuts
- Cornmeal or flour for dusting

Instructions:

1. In a large mixing bowl, combine the all-purpose flour, active dry yeast, and salt.
2. Gradually add the warm water to the dry ingredients, stirring with a wooden spoon or spatula until a shaggy dough forms.
3. Mix in the dried cranberries and chopped walnuts, ensuring they are evenly distributed throughout the dough.
4. Cover the bowl with plastic wrap or a damp cloth and let the dough rise at room temperature for about 12-18 hours. During this time, the dough will double in size and develop a lovely flavor.

5. After the first rise, preheat your oven to 450°F (230°C). Place a cast-iron Dutch oven or oven-safe pot with a lid inside the oven while it preheats.
6. Meanwhile, transfer the risen dough onto a well-floured surface. Gently shape it into a ball, adding a bit of flour as needed to prevent sticking.
7. Carefully remove the hot pot from the oven and sprinkle a bit of cornmeal or flour on the bottom to prevent sticking.
8. Place the dough ball into the preheated pot, cover it with the lid, and return it to the oven.
9. Bake the bread covered for 30 minutes. This will help create a steamy environment and a crusty exterior.
10. After 30 minutes, remove the lid, and continue baking the bread for an additional 15-20 minutes or until the crust turns golden brown.
11. Once baked, carefully remove the bread from the pot and place it on a wire rack to cool completely.
12. Allow the Cranberry Walnut Artisan Bread to cool for at least 1 hour before slicing. This resting time helps develop the bread's texture and flavor.
13. Slice and enjoy your Cranberry Walnut Artisan Bread! This rustic and flavorful bread is perfect for breakfast, as a side with soups or salads, or as a delightful snack. Store any leftovers in a bread bag or an airtight container to maintain its freshness.

Note: You can experiment with different types of nuts or dried fruits to customize the bread to your liking. Almonds, pecans, or raisins are excellent alternatives. This artisan bread is best enjoyed within a day or two of baking for optimal taste and texture.

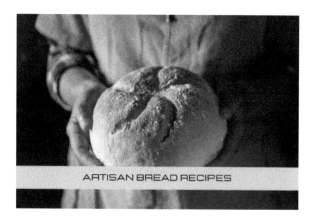

ARTISAN BREAD RECIPES

Fig and Goat Cheese Bread

Ingredients:

- 3 cups all-purpose flour
- 1 teaspoon active dry yeast
- 1 1/2 teaspoons salt
- 1 1/2 cups warm water (around 110°F or 45°C)
- 1/2 cup dried figs, chopped
- 1/2 cup crumbled goat cheese
- Cornmeal or flour for dusting

Instructions:

1. In a large mixing bowl, combine the all-purpose flour, active dry yeast, and salt.
2. Gradually add the warm water to the dry ingredients, stirring with a wooden spoon or spatula until a shaggy dough forms.
3. Mix in the chopped dried figs and crumbled goat cheese, ensuring they are evenly distributed throughout the dough.
4. Cover the bowl with plastic wrap or a damp cloth and let the dough rise at room temperature for about 12-18 hours. During this time, the dough will double in size and develop a delightful flavor.

5. After the first rise, preheat your oven to 450°F (230°C). Place a cast-iron Dutch oven or oven-safe pot with a lid inside the oven while it preheats.

6. Meanwhile, transfer the risen dough onto a well-floured surface. Gently shape it into a ball, adding a bit of flour as needed to prevent sticking.

7. Carefully remove the hot pot from the oven and sprinkle a bit of cornmeal or flour on the bottom to prevent sticking.

8. Place the dough ball into the preheated pot, cover it with the lid, and return it to the oven.

9. Bake the bread covered for 30 minutes. This will help create a steamy environment and a crusty exterior.

10. After 30 minutes, remove the lid, and continue baking the bread for an additional 15-20 minutes or until the crust turns golden brown.

11. Once baked, carefully remove the bread from the pot and place it on a wire rack to cool completely.

12. Allow the Fig and Goat Cheese Artisan Bread to cool for at least 1 hour before slicing. This resting time helps develop the bread's texture and flavor.

13. Slice and savor your Fig and Goat Cheese Artisan Bread! This unique combination of sweet figs and tangy goat cheese creates a truly delightful flavor experience. Enjoy the bread on its own, with a drizzle of honey, or paired with your favorite cheese and wine. Store any leftovers in a bread bag or an airtight container to keep it fresh.

Note: You can enhance the flavor further by adding a pinch of ground cinnamon or a sprinkle of chopped fresh rosemary to the dough. The bread is best enjoyed within a day or two of baking for optimal taste and texture.

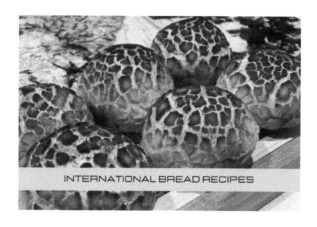

INTERNATIONAL BREAD RECIPES

Challah Bread (Jewish)

Ingredients:

- 4 cups all-purpose flour
- 1/2 cup granulated sugar
- 1 packet (2 1/4 teaspoons) active dry yeast
- 1 teaspoon salt
- 1/2 cup warm water (around 110°F or 45°C)
- 1/4 cup vegetable oil or melted unsalted butter
- 3 large eggs (plus 1 extra for egg wash)
- 1 teaspoon vanilla extract (optional)
- Poppy seeds or sesame seeds for topping (optional)

Instructions:

1. In a small bowl, combine the warm water and 1 tablespoon of sugar. Sprinkle the yeast over the water and let it sit for about 5 minutes until foamy.
2. In a large mixing bowl, whisk together the flour, remaining sugar, and salt.
3. In a separate bowl, whisk together the vegetable oil or melted butter, 3 eggs, and vanilla extract (if using).
4. Add the yeast mixture to the wet ingredients and stir to combine.

5. Gradually add the wet ingredients to the dry ingredients, mixing with a wooden spoon or spatula until a soft dough forms.
6. Transfer the dough to a floured surface and knead it for about 8-10 minutes until smooth and elastic. You can also use a stand mixer with a dough hook attachment for kneading.
7. Place the kneaded dough in a lightly oiled bowl, cover it with plastic wrap or a damp cloth, and let it rise in a warm place for about 1.5 to 2 hours until it doubles in size.
8. After the first rise, punch down the dough to release any air bubbles.
9. Divide the dough into three equal pieces. Roll each piece into a long rope, about 12 inches (30 cm) in length.
10. Lay the three ropes side by side and pinch them together at one end. Braid the ropes together, pinching the other end to seal.
11. Place the braided dough on a baking sheet lined with parchment paper. Cover it loosely with plastic wrap or a damp cloth and let it rise again for about 45 minutes to 1 hour.
12. Preheat your oven to 350°F (175°C).
13. Beat the extra egg and brush it gently over the top of the risen challah. This will give the bread a beautiful golden color when baked.
14. Optionally, sprinkle poppy seeds or sesame seeds over the top of the egg-washed challah for added texture and flavor.
15. Bake the challah in the preheated oven for 25-30 minutes or until the top is golden brown and the bread sounds hollow when tapped on the bottom.
16. Remove the challah from the oven and let it cool on a wire rack before slicing and serving.

Note: For a sweeter challah, you can add an extra tablespoon of sugar to the dough. You can also incorporate raisins, dried cranberries, or chocolate chips into the dough for a delightful twist. Challah bread is a symbol of celebration and unity in Jewish tradition, and it's sure to be a crowd-pleaser at any gathering.

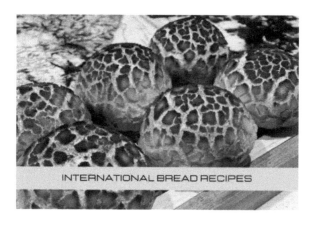

INTERNATIONAL BREAD RECIPES

Dutch Crunch Bread (Dutch)

Ingredients For the Bread:

- 4 cups bread flour
- 2 teaspoons active dry yeast
- 1 1/2 teaspoons salt
- 1 cup warm milk (around 110°F or 45°C)
- 2 tablespoons granulated sugar
- 2 tablespoons unsalted butter, softened

For the Dutch Crunch Topping:

- 1/4 cup warm water
- 1 teaspoon active dry yeast
- 1 tablespoon vegetable or olive oil
- 1 tablespoon granulated sugar
- 1/2 teaspoon salt
- 3/4 cup rice flour

Instructions:

1. In a small bowl, combine the warm milk and sugar. Sprinkle the yeast over the milk and let it sit for about 5 minutes until foamy.
2. In a large mixing bowl, whisk together the bread flour and salt.

3. Add the softened butter to the dry ingredients, followed by the yeast mixture.
4. Mix the ingredients until a dough forms. Transfer the dough to a floured surface and knead it for about 8-10 minutes until smooth and elastic. You can also use a stand mixer with a dough hook attachment for kneading.
5. Place the kneaded dough in a lightly oiled bowl, cover it with plastic wrap or a damp cloth, and let it rise in a warm place for about 1 to 1.5 hours until it doubles in size.
6. After the first rise, punch down the dough to release any air bubbles.
7. Shape the dough into a round or oval loaf, and place it on a baking sheet lined with parchment paper.
8. In a small bowl, mix the warm water, yeast, vegetable or olive oil, sugar, and salt to create the Dutch Crunch topping.
9. Add the rice flour to the wet ingredients and stir until you get a thick, smooth paste.
10. Spread the Dutch Crunch topping evenly over the top of the shaped dough, leaving a small border around the edges.
11. Cover the dough loosely with plastic wrap or a damp cloth and let it rise again for about 45 minutes to 1 hour.
12. Meanwhile, preheat your oven to 375°F (190°C).
13. Once the dough has risen again, bake the Dutch Crunch Bread in the preheated oven for 30-35 minutes or until the top is golden brown and the bread sounds hollow when tapped on the bottom.
14. Remove the bread from the oven and let it cool on a wire rack before slicing and serving.

Note: Dutch Crunch Bread is often enjoyed in the Netherlands and is known for its tiger-like appearance due to the cracked topping. The rice flour creates a crunchy and slightly sweet crust that complements the soft and fluffy interior of the bread.

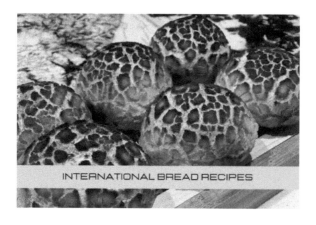

INTERNATIONAL BREAD RECIPES

Japanese Milk Bread (Japanese)

Ingredients:

- 4 cups bread flour
- 1/4 cup granulated sugar
- 2 teaspoons active dry yeast
- 1 teaspoon salt
- 1/2 cup warm milk (around 110°F or 45°C)
- 1/4 cup warm water
- 1/4 cup unsalted butter, softened
- 1/2 cup milk, at room temperature
- 1 large egg, at room temperature

Instructions:

1. In a small bowl, combine the warm milk and 1 tablespoon of sugar. Sprinkle the yeast over the milk and let it sit for about 5 minutes until foamy.
2. In a large mixing bowl, whisk together the bread flour, remaining sugar, and salt.
3. In a separate bowl, whisk together the warm water, softened butter, milk, and egg.
4. Add the yeast mixture to the wet ingredients and stir to combine.

5. Gradually add the wet ingredients to the dry ingredients, mixing with a wooden spoon or spatula until a soft dough forms.
6. Transfer the dough to a floured surface and knead it for about 8-10 minutes until smooth and elastic. You can also use a stand mixer with a dough hook attachment for kneading.
7. Place the kneaded dough in a lightly oiled bowl, cover it with plastic wrap or a damp cloth, and let it rise in a warm place for about 1 to 1.5 hours until it doubles in size.
8. After the first rise, punch down the dough to release any air bubbles.
9. Divide the dough into three equal pieces. Roll each piece into a ball and let them rest for 10 minutes.
10. Flatten each dough ball into an oval shape and then fold the sides towards the center, overlapping slightly. Roll the folded dough into a log shape.
11. Place the three dough logs side by side in a lightly greased loaf pan.
12. Cover the loaf pan loosely with plastic wrap or a damp cloth and let the dough rise again for about 45 minutes to 1 hour.
13. Meanwhile, preheat your oven to 350°F (175°C).
14. Once the dough has risen again, brush the top with a little milk for a golden finish.
15. Bake the Japanese Milk Bread in the preheated oven for 30-35 minutes or until the top is golden brown and the bread sounds hollow when tapped on the bottom.
16. Remove the bread from the oven and let it cool in the pan for a few minutes before transferring it to a wire rack to cool completely.
17. Slice and enjoy your Japanese Milk Bread! This soft and fluffy bread is perfect for sandwiches, toast, or simply with a slather of butter. Store any leftovers in an airtight container to maintain its freshness.

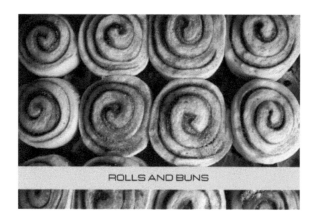

ROLLS AND BUNS

Whole Wheat Hamburger Buns

Ingredients:

- 2 cups whole wheat flour
- 1 cup all-purpose flour
- 1 packet (2 1/4 teaspoons) active dry yeast
- 1 teaspoon salt
- 1 cup warm milk (around 110°F or 45°C)
- 1/4 cup warm water
- 2 tablespoons honey or maple syrup
- 2 tablespoons unsalted butter, melted
- 1 large egg, beaten (plus 1 extra for egg wash, optional)
- Sesame seeds for topping (optional)

Instructions:

1. In a small bowl, combine the warm milk and honey (or maple syrup). Sprinkle the yeast over the milk mixture and let it sit for about 5 minutes until foamy.
2. In a large mixing bowl, whisk together the whole wheat flour, all-purpose flour, and salt.
3. Add the melted butter and beaten egg to the dry ingredients, followed by the yeast mixture.

4. Gradually add the warm water to the dough, mixing with a wooden spoon or spatula until a soft and slightly sticky dough forms.
5. Transfer the dough to a floured surface and knead it for about 8-10 minutes until smooth and elastic. You can also use a stand mixer with a dough hook attachment for kneading.
6. Place the kneaded dough in a lightly oiled bowl, cover it with plastic wrap or a damp cloth, and let it rise in a warm place for about 1 to 1.5 hours until it doubles in size.
7. After the first rise, punch down the dough to release any air bubbles.
8. Divide the dough into 8 equal pieces. Shape each piece into a smooth ball and place them on a baking sheet lined with parchment paper.
9. Flatten each dough ball slightly with the palm of your hand to create a bun shape.
10. Cover the dough balls loosely with plastic wrap or a damp cloth and let them rise again for about 30-45 minutes.
11. Meanwhile, preheat your oven to 375°F (190°C).
12. Optionally, beat an extra egg and brush it gently over the top of each risen bun. This will give the buns a beautiful golden color when baked.
13. Optionally, sprinkle sesame seeds over the egg-washed buns for added texture and flavor.
14. Bake the Whole Wheat Hamburger Buns in the preheated oven for 15-20 minutes or until the tops are golden brown and the buns sound hollow when tapped on the bottom.
15. Remove the buns from the oven and let them cool on a wire rack before slicing and serving.
16. Enjoy your homemade Whole Wheat Hamburger Buns! These wholesome buns are perfect for your favorite burgers or sandwiches. Store any leftovers in an airtight container to keep them fresh.

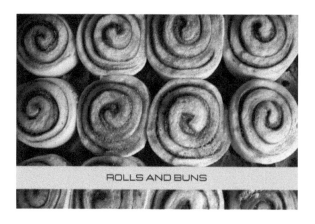

ROLLS AND BUNS

Sweet Potato Rolls

Ingredients:

- 1 cup cooked and mashed sweet potato (about 1 medium-sized sweet potato)
- 1/2 cup warm milk (around 110°F or 45°C)
- 1/4 cup unsalted butter, melted
- 1/4 cup granulated sugar
- 1 packet (2 1/4 teaspoons) active dry yeast
- 1 large egg, beaten
- 3 1/2 cups all-purpose flour
- 1 teaspoon salt

Instructions:

1. Cook the sweet potato until tender. Peel and mash it using a fork or potato masher. Measure out 1 cup of mashed sweet potato for the recipe.
2. In a small bowl, combine the warm milk and 1 tablespoon of sugar. Sprinkle the yeast over the milk mixture and let it sit for about 5 minutes until foamy.
3. In a large mixing bowl, whisk together the mashed sweet potato, melted butter, remaining sugar, and beaten egg.
4. Add the yeast mixture to the sweet potato mixture and stir to combine.

146

5. Gradually add the all-purpose flour and salt to the wet ingredients, mixing with a wooden spoon or spatula until a soft dough forms.
6. Transfer the dough to a floured surface and knead it for about 8-10 minutes until smooth and elastic. You can also use a stand mixer with a dough hook attachment for kneading.
7. Place the kneaded dough in a lightly oiled bowl, cover it with plastic wrap or a damp cloth, and let it rise in a warm place for about 1 to 1.5 hours until it doubles in size.
8. After the first rise, punch down the dough to release any air bubbles.
9. Divide the dough into 12 equal pieces. Shape each piece into a smooth ball and place them in a greased 9x13-inch baking pan or on a baking sheet lined with parchment paper.
10. Cover the dough balls loosely with plastic wrap or a damp cloth and let them rise again for about 30-45 minutes.
11. Meanwhile, preheat your oven to 375°F (190°C).
12. Optionally, brush the tops of the risen rolls with a little melted butter for a shiny finish.
13. Bake the Sweet Potato Rolls in the preheated oven for 15-20 minutes or until the tops are lightly golden brown.
14. Remove the rolls from the oven and let them cool slightly in the pan or on the baking sheet before serving.
15. Enjoy your homemade Sweet Potato Rolls! These soft and slightly sweet rolls are a delightful addition to any meal or holiday table. Serve them warm with butter or your favorite spread.

Note: Sweet Potato Rolls add a unique flavor and moisture to the classic dinner roll. The natural sweetness of the sweet potato enhances the overall taste, making these rolls a crowd-pleaser.

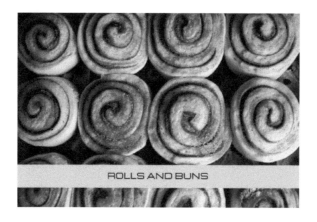

ROLLS AND BUNS

Cheddar Bacon Rolls

Ingredients:

- 3 cups all-purpose flour
- 1 packet (2 1/4 teaspoons) active dry yeast
- 1/4 cup granulated sugar
- 1 teaspoon salt
- 1/2 cup warm milk (around 110°F or 45°C)
- 1/4 cup warm water
- 1/4 cup unsalted butter, melted
- 1 large egg, beaten
- 1 cup shredded cheddar cheese
- 1/2 cup cooked and crumbled bacon (about 6-8 slices)
- 2 tablespoons chopped fresh chives (optional)
- Extra melted butter for brushing (optional)

Instructions:

1. In a small bowl, combine the warm milk and 1 tablespoon of sugar. Sprinkle the yeast over the milk mixture and let it sit for about 5 minutes until foamy.
2. In a large mixing bowl, whisk together the all-purpose flour, remaining sugar, and salt.
3. Add the melted butter and beaten egg to the dry ingredients, followed by the yeast mixture.

4. Gradually add the warm water to the dough, mixing with a wooden spoon or spatula until a soft dough forms.
5. Transfer the dough to a floured surface and knead it for about 8-10 minutes until smooth and elastic. You can also use a stand mixer with a dough hook attachment for kneading.
6. Place the kneaded dough in a lightly oiled bowl, cover it with plastic wrap or a damp cloth, and let it rise in a warm place for about 1 to 1.5 hours until it doubles in size.
7. After the first rise, punch down the dough to release any air bubbles.
8. In a separate bowl, mix together the shredded cheddar cheese, crumbled bacon, and chopped fresh chives (if using).
9. Divide the dough into 12 equal pieces. Flatten each piece into a small round disc and place a spoonful of the cheddar bacon mixture in the center.
10. Gather the edges of the dough and pinch them together to seal the filling inside, forming a ball.
11. Place the filled dough balls in a greased 9x13-inch baking pan or on a baking sheet lined with parchment paper.
12. Cover the rolls loosely with plastic wrap or a damp cloth and let them rise again for about 30-45 minutes.
13. Meanwhile, preheat your oven to 375°F (190°C).
14. Optionally, brush the tops of the risen rolls with a little melted butter for a golden finish.
15. Bake the Cheddar Bacon Rolls in the preheated oven for 15-20 minutes or until the tops are lightly golden brown and the rolls sound hollow when tapped on the bottom.
16. Remove the rolls from the oven and let them cool slightly before serving.
17. Enjoy your delicious Cheddar Bacon Rolls! These savory and cheesy rolls are perfect for brunch, picnics, or as a side dish for your favorite meals.

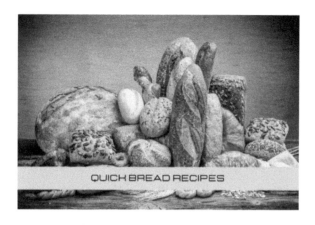

QUICH BREAD RECIPES

Orange Cranberry Bread

Ingredients:

- 2 cups all-purpose flour
- 1 cup granulated sugar
- 1 teaspoon baking powder
- 1/2 teaspoon baking soda
- 1/2 teaspoon salt
- 1/2 cup unsalted butter, melted
- 1/2 cup freshly squeezed orange juice
- Zest of one orange
- 2 large eggs, beaten
- 1 teaspoon vanilla extract
- 1 cup fresh or frozen cranberries
- Optional: 1/2 cup chopped nuts (such as walnuts or pecans)

Instructions:

1. Preheat your oven to 350°F (175°C). Grease a 9x5-inch loaf pan and set it aside.
2. In a large mixing bowl, whisk together the all-purpose flour, granulated sugar, baking powder, baking soda, and salt.

3. In a separate bowl, combine the melted butter, freshly squeezed orange juice, orange zest, beaten eggs, and vanilla extract.
4. Gradually add the wet ingredients to the dry ingredients, stirring until just combined. Be careful not to overmix.
5. Gently fold in the fresh or frozen cranberries and chopped nuts (if using).
6. Pour the batter into the prepared loaf pan, spreading it evenly.
7. Bake the Orange Cranberry Bread in the preheated oven for 55-65 minutes or until a toothpick inserted into the center comes out clean.
8. If the top of the bread starts to brown too quickly during baking, you can cover it loosely with aluminum foil to prevent over-browning.
9. Once baked, remove the bread from the oven and let it cool in the pan for about 10 minutes.
10. Carefully remove the bread from the pan and transfer it to a wire rack to cool completely.
11. Once cooled, slice and enjoy your Orange Cranberry Bread! This moist and flavorful bread is perfect for breakfast, brunch, or as a delightful afternoon treat.

Note: Orange Cranberry Bread combines the bright citrus flavor of oranges with the tartness of cranberries, creating a delicious balance of tastes. The addition of nuts adds a delightful crunch and texture. Store any leftovers in an airtight container to keep them fresh.

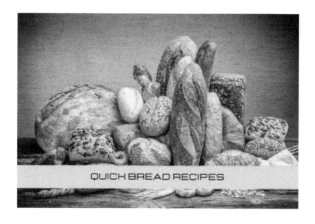

Pumpkin Chocolate Chip Bread

Ingredients:

- 1 3/4 cups all-purpose flour
- 1 teaspoon baking soda
- 1/2 teaspoon baking powder
- 1/2 teaspoon salt
- 1 teaspoon ground cinnamon
- 1/2 teaspoon ground nutmeg
- 1/4 teaspoon ground cloves
- 1 cup canned pumpkin puree
- 1/2 cup granulated sugar
- 1/2 cup packed brown sugar
- 1/2 cup vegetable oil
- 2 large eggs
- 1 teaspoon vanilla extract
- 1/4 cup milk
- 3/4 cup chocolate chips (semi-sweet or milk chocolate)

Instructions:

1. Preheat your oven to 350°F (175°C). Grease a 9x5-inch loaf pan and set it aside.
2. In a medium-sized bowl, whisk together the all-purpose flour, baking soda, baking powder, salt, ground cinnamon,

ground nutmeg, and ground cloves. Set this dry mixture aside.

3. In a large mixing bowl, combine the canned pumpkin puree, granulated sugar, brown sugar, vegetable oil, eggs, and vanilla extract. Mix until well combined.

4. Gradually add the dry ingredients to the wet ingredients, alternating with the milk, and mix until just combined. Be careful not to overmix.

5. Gently fold in the chocolate chips, distributing them evenly throughout the batter.

6. Pour the batter into the prepared loaf pan, spreading it evenly.

7. Bake the Pumpkin Chocolate Chip Bread in the preheated oven for 50-60 minutes or until a toothpick inserted into the center comes out clean.

8. If the top of the bread starts to brown too quickly during baking, you can cover it loosely with aluminum foil to prevent over-browning.

9. Once baked, remove the bread from the oven and let it cool in the pan for about 10 minutes.

10. Carefully remove the bread from the pan and transfer it to a wire rack to cool completely.

11. Once cooled, slice and enjoy your Pumpkin Chocolate Chip Bread! This moist and flavorful bread is a delightful fall treat that combines the comforting taste of pumpkin with the richness of chocolate.

Note: Pumpkin Chocolate Chip Bread is a perfect balance of autumn flavors and sweet indulgence. The chocolate chips add a delightful burst of richness to the pumpkin-spiced bread. Store any leftovers in an airtight container to keep them fresh.

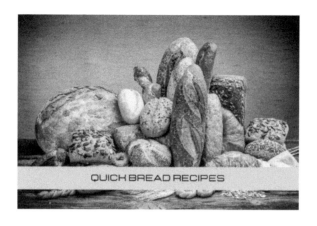

Chai Spice Bread

Ingredients:

- 2 cups all-purpose flour
- 1 teaspoon baking powder
- 1/2 teaspoon baking soda
- 1/2 teaspoon salt
- 2 teaspoons ground cinnamon
- 1 teaspoon ground ginger
- 1/2 teaspoon ground cardamom
- 1/4 teaspoon ground cloves
- 1/4 teaspoon ground nutmeg
- 1/2 cup unsalted butter, softened
- 1 cup granulated sugar
- 2 large eggs
- 1 teaspoon vanilla extract
- 1 cup plain yogurt (Greek or regular)
- 1/4 cup milk
- Optional: 1 tablespoon chai tea leaves (finely ground)
- Optional: 1/2 cup chopped nuts (almonds or walnuts)

Instructions:

1. Preheat your oven to 350°F (175°C). Grease a 9x5-inch loaf pan and set it aside.

2. In a medium-sized bowl, whisk together the all-purpose flour, baking powder, baking soda, salt, ground cinnamon, ground ginger, ground cardamom, ground cloves, and ground nutmeg. If using chai tea leaves, add them to the dry mixture.
3. In a large mixing bowl, cream the softened unsalted butter and granulated sugar until light and fluffy.
4. Add the eggs one at a time, mixing well after each addition. Stir in the vanilla extract.
5. Gradually add the dry ingredients to the butter mixture, alternating with the plain yogurt and milk. Mix until just combined. Be careful not to overmix.
6. If using chopped nuts, gently fold them into the batter.
7. Pour the batter into the prepared loaf pan, spreading it evenly.
8. Bake the Chai Spice Bread in the preheated oven for 50-60 minutes or until a toothpick inserted into the center comes out clean.
9. If the top of the bread starts to brown too quickly during baking, you can cover it loosely with aluminum foil to prevent over-browning.
10. Once baked, remove the bread from the oven and let it cool in the pan for about 10 minutes.
11. Carefully remove the bread from the pan and transfer it to a wire rack to cool completely.
12. Once cooled, slice and enjoy your Chai Spice Bread! This aromatic and flavorful bread is reminiscent of a warm cup of chai tea, making it a delightful treat for any time of the day.

Note: Chai Spice Bread offers a delightful blend of aromatic spices that evoke the comforting essence of chai tea. The addition of yogurt makes the bread moist and tender. Store any leftovers in an airtight container to keep them fresh.

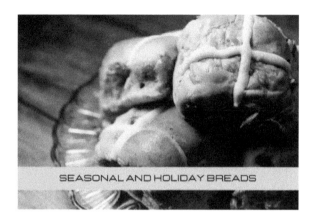

SEASONAL AND HOLIDAY BREADS

King Cake (Mardi Gras)

Ingredients For the cake dough:

- 4 cups all-purpose flour
- 1/2 cup granulated sugar
- 1 package (7g) active dry yeast
- 1 teaspoon salt
- 1/2 cup whole milk
- 1/4 cup water
- 1/2 cup unsalted butter, softened
- 4 large eggs, at room temperature
- 1 teaspoon vanilla extract
- 1 teaspoon grated lemon zest (optional)

For the filling:

- 1/2 cup packed brown sugar
- 2 teaspoons ground cinnamon
- 1/4 cup unsalted butter, softened

For the glaze:

- 2 cups powdered sugar
- 3 tablespoons whole milk
- 1/2 teaspoon vanilla extract
- Colored sugar or icing (in purple, green, and gold)

To make the cake dough, start by combining 3 cups of all-purpose flour, granulated sugar, active dry yeast, and salt in a large mixing bowl. In a small saucepan, warm the milk, water, and softened butter over low heat until the butter is melted and the mixture is warm but not boiling. Pour the warm milk mixture into the dry ingredients and mix until well combined. Add the eggs one at a time, beating well after each addition. Stir in the vanilla extract and grated lemon zest if using. Gradually add the remaining 1 cup of all-purpose flour, a little at a time, until the dough is soft and slightly sticky. Transfer the dough to a floured surface and knead it for about 5-7 minutes until it becomes smooth and elastic. Place the kneaded dough in a lightly oiled bowl, cover it with a damp kitchen towel or plastic wrap, and let it rise at room temperature for about 1 to 1.5 hours or until it doubles in size.

For the filling, mix together the packed brown sugar, ground cinnamon, and softened butter in a small bowl until you achieve a smooth paste.

To assemble and bake the King Cake, preheat your oven to 375°F (190°C) and grease a large baking sheet or line it with parchment paper. Gently deflate the risen dough and roll it out into a large rectangle, approximately 24x12 inches. Spread the filling evenly over the rolled-out dough, leaving a small border around the edges. Starting from one long side, tightly roll up the dough into a log. Shape the log into a circle and pinch the ends together to seal it, forming a ring. Place the ring on the prepared baking sheet and let it undergo the final proofing for about 20-30 minutes. Bake the King Cake in the preheated oven for about 25-30 minutes or until it turns golden brown.

For the glaze, whisk together powdered sugar, whole milk, and vanilla extract in a small bowl until you achieve a smooth glaze. Once the King Cake has cooled, drizzle the glaze over the top of the cake. To create the traditional Mardi Gras colors, sprinkle colored sugar or icing in purple, green, and gold over the glaze in alternating sections.

Enjoy this festive King Cake with family and friends, celebrating the spirit of Mardi Gras and the joyous traditions it brings.

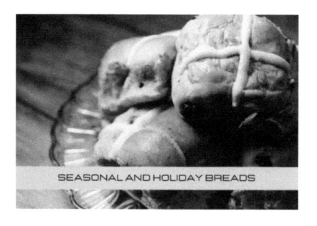

Panettone (Christmas)

Ingredients:

- 4 cups all-purpose flour
- 1/2 cup granulated sugar
- 1 packet (2 1/4 teaspoons) active dry yeast
- 1/2 cup warm milk (around 110°F or 45°C)
- 1/2 cup unsalted butter, softened
- 4 large eggs, at room temperature
- 1 teaspoon vanilla extract
- Zest of 1 orange
- Zest of 1 lemon
- 1/2 teaspoon salt
- 1/2 cup candied orange peel
- 1/2 cup candied lemon peel
- 1/2 cup golden raisins
- 1/2 cup dried currants
- Optional: 1/2 cup chopped almonds or hazelnuts
- Optional: 1/4 cup dark chocolate chips or chunks

Instructions:

1. In a small bowl, combine the warm milk and 1 tablespoon of sugar. Sprinkle the yeast over the milk mixture and let it sit for about 5 minutes until foamy.
2. In a large mixing bowl, whisk together the all-purpose flour, remaining sugar, and salt.

3. Add the softened unsalted butter, eggs, vanilla extract, orange zest, and lemon zest to the dry ingredients. Mix until the ingredients come together.
4. Gradually add the yeast mixture to the dough and mix until it becomes a smooth and elastic dough. You can use a stand mixer with a dough hook attachment for easier mixing.
5. Fold in the candied orange peel, candied lemon peel, golden raisins, dried currants, chopped almonds or hazelnuts (if using), and dark chocolate chips or chunks (if using). Mix until all the ingredients are evenly distributed throughout the dough.
6. Place the dough in a greased bowl, cover it with plastic wrap or a damp cloth, and let it rise in a warm place for about 2-3 hours or until it doubles in size.
7. After the first rise, punch down the dough to release any air bubbles.
8. Prepare a Panettone paper mold or a round baking pan by greasing it and lining the bottom with parchment paper.
9. Transfer the dough to the prepared mold or pan, shaping it into a round dome shape. Use a sharp knife to make a shallow "X" on top of the dough.
10. Cover the dough loosely with plastic wrap or a damp cloth and let it rise again for about 1-2 hours until it reaches the top of the mold or pan.
11. Meanwhile, preheat your oven to 350°F (175°C).
12. Bake the Panettone in the preheated oven for 40-50 minutes or until the top is golden brown and a toothpick inserted into the center comes out clean.
13. Once baked, remove the Panettone from the oven and let it cool in the mold or pan for about 10 minutes.
14. Carefully remove the Panettone from the mold or pan and transfer it to a wire rack to cool completely.
15. Once cooled, slice and enjoy your Panettone! This classic Italian Christmas bread is filled with delightful candied fruits, raisins, and optional nuts and chocolate, making it a true holiday indulgence.

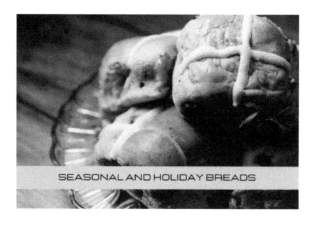

Easter Dove Bread (Easter)

Ingredients:

- 4 cups all-purpose flour
- 1/2 cup granulated sugar
- 1 packet (2 1/4 teaspoons) active dry yeast
- 1/2 cup warm milk (around 110°F or 45°C)
- 1/2 cup unsalted butter, softened
- 4 large eggs, at room temperature
- 1 teaspoon almond extract
- 1/2 teaspoon vanilla extract
- Zest of 1 lemon
- 1/2 teaspoon salt
- 1/2 cup golden raisins
- 1/4 cup sliced almonds
- Optional: 1 tablespoon orange blossom water or orange liqueur (e.g., Cointreau)
- Egg wash (1 egg beaten with 1 tablespoon milk)
- Powdered sugar for dusting

Instructions:

1. In a small bowl, combine the warm milk and 1 tablespoon of sugar. Sprinkle the yeast over the milk mixture and let it sit for about 5 minutes until foamy.
2. In a large mixing bowl, whisk together the all-purpose flour, remaining sugar, and salt.

3. Add the softened unsalted butter, eggs, almond extract, vanilla extract, and lemon zest to the dry ingredients. Mix until the ingredients come together.
4. Gradually add the yeast mixture to the dough and mix until it becomes a smooth and elastic dough. You can use a stand mixer with a dough hook attachment for easier mixing.
5. Fold in the golden raisins and sliced almonds. If using orange blossom water or orange liqueur, add it to the dough as well. Mix until all the ingredients are evenly distributed throughout the dough.
6. Place the dough in a greased bowl, cover it with plastic wrap or a damp cloth, and let it rise in a warm place for about 1-2 hours or until it doubles in size.
7. After the first rise, punch down the dough to release any air bubbles.
8. Prepare an Easter Dove Bread mold or a round baking pan by greasing it and lining the bottom with parchment paper.
9. Transfer the dough to the prepared mold or pan, shaping it into a dove-like figure. You can shape the head, wings, and tail using your hands or scissors.
10. Cover the dough loosely with plastic wrap or a damp cloth and let it rise again for about 1-2 hours until it reaches the top of the mold or pan.
11. Meanwhile, preheat your oven to 350°F (175°C).
12. Brush the risen dough with the egg wash to give it a beautiful golden color when baked.
13. Bake the Easter Dove Bread in the preheated oven for 30-40 minutes or until the top is golden brown and a toothpick inserted into the center comes out clean.
14. Once baked, remove the Easter Dove Bread from the oven and let it cool in the mold or pan for about 10 minutes.
15. Carefully remove the bread from the mold or pan and transfer it to a wire rack to cool completely.
16. Once cooled, dust the Easter Dove Bread with powdered sugar for a delightful finishing touch.
17. Display your Easter Dove Bread as a centerpiece during Easter celebrations, symbolizing peace and rebirth. Serve slices of this sweet and symbolic bread to your loved ones, embracing the spirit of Easter.

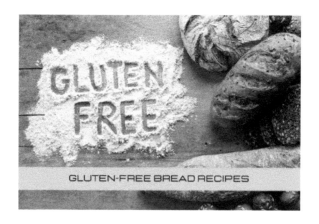

GLUTEN-FREE BREAD RECIPES

Gluten-Free Rosemary and Garlic Bread

Ingredients:

- 1 cup quinoa flour
- 1 cup gluten-free all-purpose flour
- 1/2 cup almond flour
- 1/4 cup ground flaxseed
- 1 packet (2 1/4 teaspoons) gluten-free active dry yeast
- 1 teaspoon salt
- 1 tablespoon honey or maple syrup
- 1 cup warm water (around 110°F or 45°C)
- 2 large eggs
- 2 tablespoons olive oil
- 1 teaspoon apple cider vinegar
- Optional: 1/4 cup sunflower seeds or pumpkin seeds for topping

Instructions:

1. In a small bowl, combine the warm water and honey (or maple syrup). Sprinkle the gluten-free active dry yeast over the water mixture and let it sit for about 5 minutes until foamy.

2. In a large mixing bowl, whisk together the quinoa flour, gluten-free all-purpose flour, almond flour, ground flaxseed, and salt.
3. Create a well in the center of the dry ingredients and add the foamy yeast mixture, eggs, olive oil, and apple cider vinegar.
4. Mix the wet and dry ingredients together until a smooth and thick dough forms. You can use a stand mixer with a paddle attachment for easier mixing.
5. Grease a standard-sized loaf pan (8.5 x 4.5 inches) and line it with parchment paper, leaving some excess paper on the sides for easy removal.
6. Transfer the dough to the prepared loaf pan, spreading it evenly and smoothing the top.
7. Optional: Sprinkle sunflower seeds or pumpkin seeds on top of the dough for added texture and visual appeal.
8. Cover the pan loosely with plastic wrap or a damp cloth and let the dough rise in a warm place for about 1-1.5 hours or until it doubles in size.
9. Meanwhile, preheat your oven to 375°F (190°C).
10. Once the dough has risen, remove the plastic wrap or damp cloth and bake the Gluten-Free Quinoa Bread in the preheated oven for 35-40 minutes or until the top is golden brown and the bread sounds hollow when tapped.
11. After baking, remove the bread from the oven and let it cool in the pan for about 10 minutes.
12. Carefully lift the bread out of the pan using the excess parchment paper and transfer it to a wire rack to cool completely.
13. Once cooled, slice and enjoy your Gluten-Free Quinoa Bread! This nutrient-rich and gluten-free option is perfect for those with dietary restrictions or anyone looking for a wholesome and delicious bread.

Note: Gluten-Free Quinoa Bread offers a hearty and nutritious alternative to traditional wheat-based bread. It's rich in protein, fiber, and essential nutrients from quinoa and almond flour.

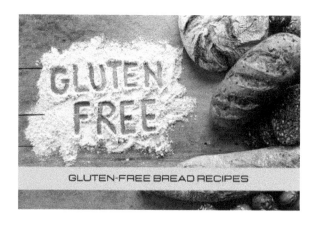

GLUTEN-FREE BREAD RECIPES

Gluten-Free Sunflower Seed Bread

Ingredients:

- 1 cup gluten-free all-purpose flour
- 1 cup almond flour
- 1/2 cup ground flaxseed
- 1/4 cup chia seeds
- 1/4 cup sunflower seeds
- 1 packet (2 1/4 teaspoons) gluten-free active dry yeast
- 1 teaspoon salt
- 1 tablespoon honey or maple syrup
- 1 cup warm water (around 110°F or 45°C)
- 2 large eggs
- 2 tablespoons olive oil
- 1 teaspoon apple cider vinegar

Instructions:

1. In a small bowl, combine the warm water and honey (or maple syrup). Sprinkle the gluten-free active dry yeast over the water mixture and let it sit for about 5 minutes until foamy.
2. In a large mixing bowl, whisk together the gluten-free all-purpose flour, almond flour, ground flaxseed, chia seeds, sunflower seeds, and salt.

3. Create a well in the center of the dry ingredients and add the foamy yeast mixture, eggs, olive oil, and apple cider vinegar.
4. Mix the wet and dry ingredients together until a smooth and thick dough forms. You can use a stand mixer with a paddle attachment for easier mixing.
5. Grease a standard-sized loaf pan (8.5 x 4.5 inches) and line it with parchment paper, leaving some excess paper on the sides for easy removal.
6. Transfer the dough to the prepared loaf pan, spreading it evenly and smoothing the top.
7. Optional: Sprinkle additional sunflower seeds on top of the dough for added texture and visual appeal.
8. Cover the pan loosely with plastic wrap or a damp cloth and let the dough rise in a warm place for about 1-1.5 hours or until it doubles in size.
9. Meanwhile, preheat your oven to 375°F (190°C).
10. Once the dough has risen, remove the plastic wrap or damp cloth and bake the Gluten-Free Sunflower Seed Bread in the preheated oven for 35-40 minutes or until the top is golden brown and the bread sounds hollow when tapped.
11. After baking, remove the bread from the oven and let it cool in the pan for about 10 minutes.
12. Carefully lift the bread out of the pan using the excess parchment paper and transfer it to a wire rack to cool completely.
13. Once cooled, slice and enjoy your Gluten-Free Sunflower Seed Bread! This nutty and wholesome option is perfect for those with dietary restrictions or anyone looking for a nutritious and flavorful bread.

Note: Gluten-Free Sunflower Seed Bread offers a delightful blend of nutty flavors and is packed with healthy fats, fiber, and essential nutrients from almond flour, flaxseed, chia seeds, and sunflower seeds.

Troubleshooting Guide:

Common issues and how to fix them in bread machine baking.

Bread machine baking is generally straightforward, but occasionally, you might encounter some issues. Don't worry! With a few adjustments and troubleshooting, you can overcome these challenges and achieve perfectly baked loaves. Here's a guide to common problems and their solutions:

1. Flat or Sunken Bread:

Possible Causes: Insufficient yeast, expired yeast, too much liquid, too much sugar, or opening the lid during baking.

Solution: Check yeast expiration date and use fresh yeast. Ensure proper measuring of yeast, liquid, and sweeteners. Avoid opening the bread machine during baking as it disrupts the baking process.

2. Dense and Heavy Bread:

Possible Causes: Too much flour, insufficient yeast, expired yeast, not enough rising time, or using old baking powder or baking soda.

Solution: Measure flour accurately using the spoon-and-level method. Use fresh yeast and ensure the dough has ample time to rise. Check the expiration date of baking powder or baking soda and replace if needed.

166

3. Bread Collapsed or Caved In:

Possible Causes: Too much liquid, too much sugar, too much yeast, or overproofing the dough.

Solution: Double-check ingredient measurements, especially liquid and sugar. Reduce the amount of yeast as excess yeast can cause overexpansion and collapse. Avoid overproofing the dough; follow recommended rising times.

4. Uneven Rising or Gummy Texture:

Possible Causes: Uneven distribution of ingredients, inaccurate measurements, too much liquid, too much sugar, or opening the lid during baking.

Solution: Mix ingredients thoroughly to ensure even distribution. Measure ingredients accurately. Adjust liquid and sugar amounts as needed. Avoid opening the bread machine during the baking cycle.

5. Bread Sticks to the Pan:

Possible Causes: Insufficient greasing of the bread pan or using an old, scratched pan.

Solution: Make sure to grease the bread pan properly before adding ingredients. Consider replacing old, scratched pans.

6. Crust Too Dark or Burnt:

Possible Causes: Bread machine setting for crust color is too dark, too much sugar in the recipe, or overbaking.

Solution: Adjust the bread machine setting for crust color to a lighter option. Reduce the amount of sugar in the recipe. Check the bread during baking and remove it promptly once done.

7. Bread Doesn't Rise:

Possible Causes: Inactive yeast (expired or too old), liquid too hot or too cold, or using non-fresh ingredients.

Solution: Use fresh yeast and ensure it's activated by dissolving it in warm water (around 110°F/43°C) with a pinch of sugar before adding to the machine. Check liquid temperature; it should be warm but not too hot or cold.

8. Overly Dry Bread:

Possible Causes: Too much flour, too little liquid, or the bread machine setting requires adjustments.

Solution: Check the flour measurement and use the spoon-and-level method. Adjust the liquid amount if the dough appears too dry. Experiment with different bread machine settings, such as a different loaf size or crust color.

Remember, troubleshooting is a normal part of the baking process. Be patient and open to adjusting recipes or methods as needed. With practice, you'll become a bread machine baking expert, and your kitchen will be filled with the delightful aroma of freshly baked bread!

Tip and Tricks

Creative ideas for customizing recipes.

Bread machine baking provides an excellent foundation for creating delicious loaves, and with a touch of creativity, you can transform basic recipes into extraordinary bread masterpieces. Here are some tips and tricks to customize your bread machine recipes and elevate your baking game:

1. Mix Up the Flour: Experiment with different flours to add unique flavors and textures to your bread. Try incorporating whole wheat, rye, spelt, or even gluten-free flour for alternative options.
2. Enhance with Herbs and Spices: Add a burst of flavor by incorporating herbs and spices into your dough. Rosemary, thyme, garlic, cinnamon, and cardamom are just a few options to tantalize your taste buds.
3. Go Nutty and Seedy: Add depth and crunch to your bread by mixing in various nuts and seeds. Walnuts, almonds, sunflower seeds, and flaxseeds are excellent choices.
4. Sweeten the Deal: Sweet bread varieties are always a hit. Consider adding dried fruits, such as raisins, cranberries, or apricots, as well as chocolate chips or shredded coconut for a delightful treat.
5. Cheese Please: For savory indulgence, incorporate shredded cheddar, parmesan, or feta cheese into your dough. Cheese-filled breads are perfect for pairing with soups or enjoyed as a standalone delight.

169

6. Play with Fillings: Roll out your dough and experiment with different fillings for swirl breads. Cinnamon sugar, pesto, Nutella, or even savory options like spinach and feta can take your bread to a new level.
7. Make It Zesty: For a burst of citrusy goodness, add lemon or orange zest to your dough. The tangy flavor complements sweet and savory bread alike.
8. Add a Healthy Twist: Boost the nutritional value by including ingredients like grated carrots, mashed sweet potatoes, or pureed pumpkin. Not only do they add nutrients, but they also contribute to the bread's moisture.
9. Go Savory with Onion and Garlic: Sautéed onions or roasted garlic can add a savory kick to your bread, making it an excellent accompaniment to soups or sandwiches.
10. Experiment with Fillings: Get creative with stuffed bread. Create pockets of goodness with fillings like spinach and feta, ham and cheese, or even pizza toppings.
11. Create Stunning Bread Designs: Use the dough setting of your bread machine to knead and shape the dough for artistic bread designs. Braids, twists, and decorative shapes add a touch of elegance to your loaves.
12. Explore Ethnic Flavors: Take inspiration from different cuisines and explore international flavors. Incorporate ingredients like curry powder for an Indian-inspired bread or olives and oregano for a Mediterranean twist.

With these tips and tricks, the possibilities for customizing your bread machine recipes are endless. Don't be afraid to get creative, experiment, and embrace your inner bread artist. Let your imagination guide you as you craft an array of uniquely delicious breads that will impress and delight your family and guests.

Ways to adjust recipes for dietary preferences.

Adjusting bread machine recipes to cater to specific dietary preferences is a wonderful way to ensure that everyone can enjoy the deliciousness of freshly baked bread. Here are some ways to adapt recipes for various dietary needs:

1. Gluten-Free Option:

Replace regular flour with a gluten-free flour blend or a combination of gluten-free flours like rice flour, almond flour, and tapioca flour.

Add xanthan gum (or another suitable binder) to improve the bread's texture and rise in the absence of gluten.

Use gluten-free oats or quinoa flakes for added texture and nutrition in specialty breads.

2. Dairy-Free Option:

Substitute dairy milk with plant-based milk alternatives like almond milk, soy milk, oat milk, or coconut milk.

Replace butter with dairy-free alternatives like vegan butter or coconut oil.

3. Egg-Free Option:

Use a "flax egg" (1 tablespoon ground flaxseed mixed with 3 tablespoons water) or "chia egg" (1 tablespoon chia seeds mixed with 3 tablespoons water) as a binder in place of eggs. Commercial egg replacers or unsweetened applesauce can also work as egg substitutes.

4. Vegan-Friendly Option:

Combine the adjustments mentioned for dairy-free and egg-free options to make the recipe completely vegan.

Check the ingredient list for any animal-derived products like honey, and replace them with plant-based alternatives like maple syrup or agave nectar.

5. Lower Sugar Option:

Reduce the amount of sugar or sweetener in the recipe. For mildly sweet loaves, use a fraction of the recommended sugar or substitute with natural sweeteners like applesauce or mashed bananas.

6. Low-Carb or Keto Option:

Replace traditional flours with almond flour or coconut flour for a lower-carb alternative.

Utilize low-carb sweeteners like erythritol, stevia, or monk fruit to maintain sweetness while reducing sugar content.

7. High-Fiber Option:

Add ingredients like ground flaxseed, chia seeds, or wheat bran to boost fiber content.

Incorporate whole grains like oats or quinoa for added fiber and nutrition.

8. Nut-Free Option:

Replace nuts with seeds like sunflower seeds or pumpkin seeds for a nut-free crunch.

Use seed butters (e.g., sunflower seed butter) instead of nut butters.

9. Reduced Sodium Option:

Decrease the amount of salt in the recipe. A small amount of salt is necessary for flavor, but it can often be reduced without significantly affecting the bread's quality.

Always make sure to double-check the ingredients you use to ensure they are suitable for the intended dietary preferences or restrictions. Customizing recipes to meet various dietary needs opens up a world of possibilities, allowing everyone to enjoy the pleasure of homemade bread that aligns with their individual preferences and requirements.

Ingredient substitution suggestions.

When baking with a bread machine, you may encounter situations where you need to substitute certain ingredients due to dietary preferences, allergies, or simply because you don't have a specific item on hand. Here are some useful ingredient substitution suggestions to help you navigate such situations:

1. All-Purpose Flour Substitutions:

Whole Wheat Flour: For a healthier alternative, replace a portion or all of the all-purpose flour with whole wheat flour. Keep in mind that whole wheat flour may require slightly more liquid in the recipe.

Bread Flour: If a recipe calls for bread flour but you have only all-purpose flour, you can use it as a substitute. However, the bread may be slightly less chewy.

2. Gluten-Free Flour Substitutions:

Gluten-Free Flour Blend: When a recipe calls for a specific gluten-free flour, you can use a pre-made gluten-free flour blend as a one-to-one replacement for wheat-based flours.

Almond Flour: Almond flour can be used in some gluten-free recipes to add a nutty flavor and a delicate texture.

3. Sugar Substitutions:

Honey: Swap granulated sugar with an equal amount of honey for a natural sweetener with added moisture and flavor.

Maple Syrup: Substitute granulated sugar with an equal amount of maple syrup, which also contributes a unique taste to the bread.

Agave Nectar: Use agave nectar as an alternative to sugar, especially for vegan or plant-based recipes.

4. Dairy Substitutions:

Plant-Based Milk: Replace cow's milk with plant-based milk alternatives like almond milk, soy milk, oat milk, or coconut milk for a dairy-free option.

Dairy-Free Yogurt: In recipes that call for yogurt, use dairy-free yogurt made from soy, almond, or coconut.

5. Egg Substitutions:

Flaxseed or Chia Seed Eggs: To replace eggs as a binder, mix 1 tablespoon of ground flaxseed or chia seeds with 3 tablespoons of water and let it sit for a few minutes to form a gel-like consistency.

Applesauce: Unsweetened applesauce can be used as a substitute for eggs to add moisture to the bread.

6. Butter and Oil Substitutions:

Coconut Oil: Swap butter or vegetable oil with coconut oil for a healthier alternative with a mild coconut flavor.

Applesauce: Use unsweetened applesauce as a substitute for oil to reduce the fat content in the bread.

7. Nut and Seed Substitutions:

Nuts and Seeds: If you have allergies to certain nuts or seeds, feel free to omit or replace them with safe alternatives in recipes that call for them.

8. Spice and Herb Substitutions:

Customize Flavors: Experiment with different herbs and spices to suit your taste preferences. For example, if you don't have a specific spice on hand, try a complementary one that you enjoy.

Always remember that substitutions can alter the final texture and taste of the bread, so it's best to experiment with smaller batches or use well-tested substitution recommendations. By exploring ingredient swaps, you'll discover endless possibilities for customizing recipes and creating bread that perfectly suits your preferences and dietary needs.

Brean Machine Cookbook

@2023 Alessia Sofia Ferrari